T I P - A - D A Y   G U I D E   F O R
Healthy Living

365 Simple Ways to Improve Your Health,
One Day at a Time

Melanie Douglass

DESERET
BOOK

Salt Lake City, Utah

The advice and recommendations presented in this book are intended to be used as an educational resource and to assist readers in making informed decisions. This book is not intended to replace the advice of a medical professional. Always consult with your physician before implementing these or any exercise and nutrition recommendations. The author and the publisher disclaim any liability arising from directly or indirectly using this book.

All nutrient information was collected from food labels and the USDA Agricultural Research Service Nutrient Database for Standard Reference, Release 18. Nutrient information was accurate at the time of publication.

Photos by Dunker Imaging, Inc. 2006

Library of Congress Cataloging-in-Publication Data

Douglass, Melanie.
  Tip-a-day guide for healthy living : 365 simple ways to improve your health, one day at a time / Melanie Douglass.
    p. cm.
  ISBN-10 1-59038-702-3 (pbk.)
  ISBN-13 978-1-59038-702-3 (pbk.)
  1. Health—Miscellanea. 2. Nutrition—Miscellanea. 3. Diet—Miscellanea.
  4. Exercise—Miscellanea. I. Title.
  RA776.5.D68 2007
  613.7—dc22   2006033197

Printed in the United States of America
R. R. Donnelley and Sons, Crawfordsville, IN

10   9   8   7   6   5   4   3   2

TIP-A-DAY GUIDE FOR
Healthy Living

*"Now ye may suppose
that this is foolishness in me;
but behold I say unto you,
that by small and simple things
are great things brought to pass;
and small means in many instances
doth confound the wise."*

—ALMA 37:6

ACKNOWLEDGMENTS

There are many remarkable people who have been powerful examples and influences in my life, literally guiding me along this path, helping me to find practical and doable ways to make good health happen one day at a time. From intelligent professors, effective teachers, and fabulous employers to wonderful aunts, loving family members, and inspiring friends, these people have *continually* supported me, influenced me, and educated me. Thanks to all.

In addition, there are a few who made unique contributions to my effort to learn healthy living and then translate my understandings into this book. I literally could not have accomplished this task without their support:

My husband, Danny, for being there at all times and in everything I attempt to do.

My children, for always making me feel truly happy and for giving me the daily determination to do just a *little bit better.*

My parents and in-laws, whose profound, positive impact on my life is beyond measure.

The people at Deseret Book, including Jana Erickson and Jay Parry, for their patience, valuable feedback, and outstanding work.

And Chris Dunker of Dunker Imaging, for *always* taking the perfect photo.

INTRODUCTION

22,464. That's the number of calories you could save each year by simply eating *unbuttered* toast. It's a seemingly insignificant sacrifice that brings very significant results.

If I told you that you had to "eat less and move more" to reclaim your health, would you be shocked? Would you think, "Wow, that is really revolutionary!" Not likely. Most of us know what needs to be done to improve our health. We know those familiar "eat less, move more" words very well *on paper*. And it seems so easy. It *should* work. But it doesn't. We have too much food, too little reason to move, and a society too focused on telling us what's wrong with our bodies instead of what's right. The problem isn't *understanding* what needs to be done—it's finding practical ways to make it happen in day-to-day life.

Daily efforts to improve our health require us to address not only how much we eat or exercise, but how we *think*. And reprogramming our thought process doesn't happen overnight; those thoughts are complex, interrelated, and embedded deep in our subconscious minds. Telling ourselves to just "Stop it!"—referring to eating the wrong things or being too sedentary—doesn't work. If it did, we wouldn't be struggling with such issues.

So let's take this one baby step at a time. By experimenting with "one tip a day," you're going to find 30, 130, or 330 things that work for you, your life, and your circumstances. These very focused actions will help to create a mental focus on health that maybe wasn't there before. You'll likely find yourself making other healthy choices along the way; you'll feel better, improve your health, lose weight, improve your self-esteem, and keep your sanity.

Always know that you're not alone in your search for better health. Longing to feel vibrant, healthy, and lean is something worth valiantly fighting for—you deserve to feel that way and so does your family. But in our society, "better health" has become almost mythical. We tend to think we need some radical new diet plan, a magic pill, or a breakthrough potion to help us find good health. We continue to reach, but the latest gimmicks never come through for us.

The reality is that there's no one right way for everybody to improve their health. There is no single, unique blueprint for all mankind. The reality is that different methods work on different days, based on the situation, the surroundings, and your mood. So in this book I give you a smorgasbord of different ideas. This is it, the end of the rainbow: a huge well of tips to help you make good health happen year round. Just pick one thing you can do *today.* You can go in any order. Start with Tip #365 if you want. If a tip works for you—and you make a mental connection with the philosophy—then you'll naturally want to do it again and incorporate it into your lifestyle.

The only rule is that you have to choose one—and really do it! (By the way, that's the most important part: these tips require *action*!) Don't worry, you don't have to start drinking wheat-grass juice next week and run a marathon after that. I've been there with you, dealing with food and exercise issues in real life—out in the front lines—in grocery stores, movie theatres, restaurants, fast-food chains, sporting events, airports, and much more. That's why I've tried hard to make each and every tip practical and doable in the real world. There's so much to do and so little time—you can't do it all. But you can do something. That's why some days you can perfectly control your calorie intake or cook healthy, some days you can exercise more efficiently, some days you can get eight hours of sleep—and some days you don't do a single thing right. It's called balance.

Which reminds me—22,464 calories equals *six pounds* of body weight. That's weight you could gain, lose, or *not gain* based on just one of your day-to-day decisions. And there are 364 other great tips presented in this book. Give up something good for something better. Profound changes often occur from seemingly "little" things. Don't believe me? Give it a try.

Appreciate Your Body

Your Body Is Divine . . .

With 206 sturdy bones,

more than 650 dynamic muscles,

12 perfectly synchronized organ systems,

and over 10,000,000,000,000,000 (trillion) life-giving human cells.

Your Body Is Miraculous . . .

Every day your heart beats over 103,000 times,

your respiratory system powers 25,920 breaths,

your body produces a consistent 98.6 degrees of heat,

and your body produces almost 200 billion new blood cells each

day.*

And That's Just the Beginning . . .

Every day your mind, body, and spirit work together to give you the fortitude to fulfill family, church, work, and community obligations. You take good care of everyone else; it's time to take care of you.

Make a promise to yourself—right now—that you will appreciate your body as the precious gift from God it was meant to be. Satan is jealous of your physical body because he doesn't have one—and he'll continually try to seduce you to abuse, neglect, and despise yours. Don't let him.

---

*Source: Mark D. Scott, *The Amazing Red Blood Cell.* See www.bloodservices.ca 10/2/06.

Keep a Food Journal

Keep a food journal for today. Write down what you eat, how much you eat, what time and why you ate the food. If the journaling goes well today, try to keep your food journal for a week or two—it will help you see where your health habits may need improvement. It's too easy to forget about the little snacks and nibbles that happen throughout the day. A handful here and handful there can add up to hundreds of extra calories you don't even realize you're eating.

You don't need a fancy journal to keep track of your food intake for a day. Grab a piece of scratch paper, use your day planner, or find an old notebook that you can tote around for a day.

Here's a sample layout for your food journal:

Food Item	Amount	Time of Day	Reason for Eating
Pretzels	2 large handfuls	3:30 P.M.	I was bored

Out of Sight, Out of Mind

Keep sweet treats and salty snacks out of sight today. But just to clarify: these are not forbidden foods. Rather they are "occasional" foods that turn into "everyday" foods when they're sitting in plain sight, tempting us day after day. So place these types of foods in the highest cupboard—like the one high above the fridge. If you have to actually grab a chair to reach a certain snack food, it will be ridiculously inconvenient to overindulge.

Then open your fridge and move anything that's a sweet or salty snack to the very back, making it hard to reach and out of sight. Remove any candy dishes or bags of treats from your sight. The simple rule of "out of sight, out of mind" means you can still enjoy those snack foods once in a while (as you should!) but not multiple times every day.

Use Those Abs!

Stomach crunches aren't the only way to strengthen and tone your abs. You can work your abs in almost every activity you do: sitting, standing, cleaning, typing, and even lying down! Strong abs will protect your back, reduce the incidence of back pain, and improve your posture, stability, and strength in everyday activities.

Contract your abdominal muscles as much as you can today. Start right now. Squeeze your abs and pull your belly button *in* toward your spine. Think of your abs like a sponge—you want to squeeze all the water out. To increase the contraction, bring your ribs downward about one inch toward your hip bones. Hold the contraction as long as you can. Go through this "stop-contract-and-hold" process at least ten times today.

You're likely to forget as your busy day goes on (you've probably already stopped squeezing your abs from just a few sentences ago), so do something to help you remember: wear a ring on a different finger, wear a different bracelet, wear a different belt to remind you of your goal. Okay, get going—contract those abs tight!

Sugar: Not So Sweet

Make a point to learn about sugar today. Read the nutrition facts label (if available) and look at the grams of sugar for everything you eat. Start with this important fact: four grams of sugar equal one teaspoon of sugar.

For example: A common 2-cup bowl of (not to mention any names!) Fruity Circles has 24 grams of sugar, which equals 6 teaspoons of sugar. A 20-ounce bottle of soda has 66 grams of sugar, which equals 17 teaspoons of sugar. Yikes!

Some foods have natural sugar, and some have the common table sugar added. Foods like milk and fruits have natural sugars, but they also have fiber, vitamins, minerals, antioxidants, and disease-fighting phyto-chemicals. Foods with added sugars—like treats such as soda, fruit drinks, fruit snacks, pudding, ice cream, fruited yogurts, and most snack foods—generally do not contain these nutrients. Try to eat no more than ten teaspoons of added sugar today. (That's the recommendation for healthy living, but we usually consume much more than that. You'll see.)

The Eat-Less-in-the-Evening Trick

Brush your teeth right after dinner tonight. You'll be less inclined to eat after brushing your teeth because (1) the disinfectant-like taste in your mouth ruins your appetite for snack foods; (2) even if you do cave in and eat food it won't taste good because of the aftertaste; and (3) you won't want to have to go and brush your teeth again before bed.

If dinner is served early and you find yourself needing a little something extra, brush your teeth right after eating a *sensible* evening snack (like fruit, nuts, raw veggies, a glass of milk, or a handful of whole-grain cereal). It's best to keep your after-dinner snack choices healthy since you won't be burning a lot of calories as you sleep through the night. But for those of us who are tempted to eat anything with fat, sugar, or salt late in the evening, this little trick does wonders.

Start Your Morning Right

Go to bed half an hour earlier tonight. Then wake yourself up thirty minutes earlier and squeeze in a revitalizing thirty-minute walk or workout. Mornings are the perfect time for exercise. You'll feel more energetic within the first five minutes of exercise, and that energy will keep you going throughout the day. Additionally, the increased blood flow delivers oxygen and nutrients throughout your body, and you'll have a better ability to focus and concentrate as you go about your day. You're more likely to be active on a consistent basis if you can get your workout done first thing in the morning. We've all learned the hard way that other priorities will always come up and, more often than not, exercise will eventually get bumped off of your priority list as your busy day gets even busier.

If you're worried about missing the late evening news, realize that you can catch the news morning, noon, early evening, and night. Try watching the morning news while you work out. Or listen to news on the radio or check news and weather on your local news website.

The Power of Green

Eat something leafy and green today.

When it comes to greens, there's much more than plain, old iceberg lettuce. Try one of these greens today:

- Arugula
- Endive
- Watercress
- Kale
- Spinach
- Romaine lettuce

These foods are powerful foods; they make vibrant nutrient-packed salads, add color and flavor to sandwiches, and serve up unbeatable nutrition. You can also steam or boil leafy greens and add them to main dishes. And yes, the "cooking" of greens is healthy! One cup of *raw* spinach has 30 mg of calcium, whereas one cup of *cooked* spinach has about 250 mg of calcium—that's almost as much calcium in a glass of milk! It doesn't mean you should eat *only* cooked greens. It just means you should eat some cooked and some raw; each food state offers unique benefits.

If you have no access to leafy greens today, add them to your grocery list right now.

"Why Doesn't Healthy Food Taste Good?"

My husband brought up an interesting point one day. He said, "If fruits, vegetables, and whole grains really are so great—and God has told us they are healthiest for us—then why didn't he make them taste better?"

I have a theory on this. Satan works hard every day to deceive us. Infiltrating our food supply with foods swimming in calories, fat, sodium, and sugar is a subtle yet powerful way to get us down. Fruits, vegetables, and whole grains *did* taste superior to any other food at one time—before our taste buds were introduced to the food of the twenty-first century.

So think about that today. Give credit where credit is due. Satan has succeeded at creating a relentless pressure to eat; he wants you to eat a bunch of junk that provides temporal satisfaction only. He is jealous of your physical body and wants you to degrade yours. The more advanced our food supply becomes, the more power he has to tempt you. So don't let him. You are stronger and better than he is. Let *that* give you the willpower and determination to make the healthier choice today.

New Exercise Move: An Anywhere, Anytime Squat

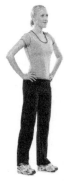

Learn how to do a basic squat today. A squat is a great exercise that targets your hips, gluteals, and thighs. This is a basic exercise that can be done anywhere at any time—no equipment necessary.

Proper form is important. Stand with your feet shoulder width apart and your toes pointing forward. Press your shoulders down and back, like you are pinching your shoulder blades together, and pull your belly button in toward your spine. Now press your hips back and down like you are going to sit into a chair. Extend your arms, reaching forward. Push your weight through your heels as you lower down. To protect your knees, make sure you keep your knees over your shoelaces—don't let your knees jet forward past your toes.

Go down as far as you are comfortable, but *don't* ever go lower than a 90-degree bend at the knees. That's too deep and can lead to injury for most people.

Keep the movement slow and controlled. Two counts down and two counts up. March in place for one to three minutes to warm up; then try to do ten to twenty repetitions. Rest and repeat the exercise ten to twenty more times. Three sets of ten to twenty reps every day will help to strengthen and tone your lower body.

Baking for Busy Moms: Wholesome Whole-Wheat Bread

Try this simple and delicious homemade whole-wheat bread recipe. (I'm not the best cook, so if I can do it, you can, too!)

Homemade Whole-Wheat Bread

Stir the following together and set aside:

¼ cup warm water

1 tablespoon yeast

1 teaspoon sugar

In a separate bowl, mix together:

2½ cups hot water

¼ cup canola oil

¼ cup sugar

¾ tablespoon salt

3 cups whole-wheat flour

Add yeast mixture and mix for 5 to 10 minutes.

Next add:

½ cup potato flakes (optional)

3 to 4 more cups whole-wheat flour

Mix until the dough pulls away from the sides of the bowl.

Divide the dough into 2 loaves and place in bread pans coated with cooking spray. Let the dough rise until it doubles in size; if you're in a hurry, let it rise for about 30 minutes. Bake at 350 degrees for 20 to 25 minutes, until golden brown. Makes 2 loaves.

Drink Up!

Juice, chocolate milk, lemonade, bottled fruit-flavored drinks, soda pop, hot chocolate, smoothies, even milk. These beverages all have two things in common: calories and sugar. They all supply at least 100 calories per cup (some have more). And nobody drinks just one cup at a time.

So let's say you drink a 12-ounce bottle of juice for breakfast, a 32-ounce soda for lunch, and an 8-ounce glass of chocolate milk for dinner. You just added more than 700 calories to your day! (It's possible to lose 1 to 1½ pounds per week *just* by cutting calorie-laden beverages out of your diet.)

Drink water with every meal today. It doesn't matter if you eat at a fast food restaurant, a fancy sit-down restaurant, or at home—wherever and whatever you eat, make sure you have a tall glass of water by your side.

There's No Rush

Most diet programs come with a time limit. Twelve-week, six-week, thirty-day, ten-day, even twenty-four-hour quick-fix programs are rampant in society today. The creators of such popular programs may not intend for it to feel like there's a "time limit." But that's what it feels like to you—the person attempting to lose weight in a specified time period decided upon by a complete stranger. Quick-fix programs train us to completely remodel our health habits in a short period of time—getting our adrenaline pumping and creating that "do it *all* now" mindset. The immense pressure makes it all too easy to say, "I'm behind. Just forget the whole thing. I can't do this."

Set a goal today to keep doing what I *hope* you're doing by reading this book. Take it one day at a time and one step at a time; work on small things that add up to make a big difference. There's no rush. It's not a race. You're working on a *permanent* shift in how you think, feel, and function in everyday life. It's not going to happen overnight.

The Truth about the First Two Weeks of Change

Handy new health book? Check. New workout shoes? Check. Fridge stocked with "health" foods? Check.

How many times have you or someone you know been in this position? All the tools are in your hands. You're motivated, inspired, and eager to change your life—forever, right? Not so fast.

You have to accept the natural ebb and flow of life. Changing health habits is never easy—you'll have good days and bad. Accept and prepare yourself for it. You might eat a new food that tastes like dirt (at first). You might go to aerobics class and think you're in a torture chamber. And you know what? It's okay. Accept the fact that you won't automatically love every new thing you try. You might hate the first two weeks of trying something new. But when the potential payoff for your efforts is life-changing, you've got to give it some time. In two weeks you might be able to stand it, and in four weeks you might love it. You never know until you try.

Say Good-bye to Boring Walks

If you have access to a treadmill, an outdoor road, a mall, indoor track, or even a yard that allows you to walk laps around the house, you can do this simple walking workout! And this isn't a drab walking experience. This is a time-flying efficient workout that's good for you—mind, body, and spirit.

Today you need to go for a thirty-minute interval-training walk. The interval training part is what makes it fun. Here's how you do it:

1. Start with three to five minutes of walking at a moderate pace to warm up.
2. Next, walk as fast as you can, taking short quick steps and pumping your arms, for one minute.
3. Then go back to a challenging but doable pace for one minute.
4. Repeat the cycle for twenty-four minutes (about twelve times).
5. Cool down with an easy walk for three to five minutes.

That's it. Work hard—and push it—for one minute. Then work at a moderate pace for one minute. Then repeat, repeat, repeat, and walk your way to better health!

Burn Calories with Good Posture

What is good posture? Take a moment to notice how you are sitting right now. Okay, now try this:

1. Pull your belly button in toward your spine and contract your abdominal muscles.
2. Bring your shoulders down and back, like you are going to pinch your shoulder blades together.
3. Bring your head back so that your ears line up with your shoulders.

Comfy? Probably not. Most of us have terrible posture. We aren't used to sitting up straight and it likely feels incredibly awkward. But using your muscles to hold good posture not only burns more calories, but it can also improve your muscle balance, which optimizes muscular movements and reduces pain and injury.

You're going to need a reminder for this one. Put one of your rings on a different finger or wear something on your wrist you don't normally wear. This will remind you to sit, stand, and walk in good posture today.

The Power of Positive

Have you ever uttered the words, "I'm too fat," "I'm too out of shape," "I'm too flabby," or other negative, nonproductive thoughts? If you're human, the answer is probably a resounding "yes!" Most of us are pretty harsh when it comes to our physical attributes. We forget about all the good things we do and pick at ourselves by saying things to ourselves we would never say to someone else. And what good does it do? Does it motivate you to go do something positive? Not likely. Picking on yourself gets you down, making you think and do negative things like "Oh, forget it. I'm a fat slob and there's no hope, so I'll just eat this whole pint of ice cream."

So today your job is to be positive about yourself. Don't say anything negative about your physical shape or size. Think about your positive attributes today. Those good attributes deserve to be taken care of. That's the motivation to make the healthier choices.

Get a Grip on Portions

I know, you're busy. You don't have time to measure everything you eat. But controlling portion size is a key and vital component in achieving good health. So practice this quick and efficient method for eyeballing proper food portions—or your health will truly suffer.

Today, you need to acknowledge that there are ridiculously large portions of food tempting you on every corner. Therefore, make sure everything you eat today is a sensible portion. Every serving of a food item should *fit in the palm of your hand.* Imagine a serving of pasta that fits in the palm of your hand; or a serving of brown rice, an apple, a roll, a piece of meat, a handful of pretzels—all of these servings should easily fit in the palm of your hand. A serving of any beverage is just eight ounces—that's less than a can of soda. So to eyeball the proper beverage portion size, visualize a can of soda that's three-fourths full. If you ever question a portion size, take a moment to check the nutrition facts label.

Based on the new USDA Food Guide Pyramid, the average adult needs about two cups of fruit, two to three cups of vegetables, three servings of whole grains, five to six ounces of lean protein, and three cups of dairy each day. Visit www.mypyramid.gov for customized recommendations based on your gender, age, and activity level.

Find a Workout Buddy

It makes perfect sense. Find a friend to work out with and you'll stick to your goal to take better care of your body. A friend, a family member, a child who counts on you, a personal trainer, or a neighbor—any of these people can help you work out consistently, benefiting both you and your buddy because you both get to reap the payoffs of good old-fashioned exercise.

Today, schedule a thirty- to sixty-minute workout with a workout buddy—someone you can count on. Make a commitment to go for a walk, a run, or a bike ride, to play a game of tennis or other sport, or to try an in-home aerobics video together. The exercise will be more fun, time will go by more quickly, and you'll likely work more effectively. More important, you'll keep your commitment to yourself to get at least thirty minutes of heart-pumping exercise that your body desperately needs today.

Listen to Your Body

Today you need to be a very conscientious eater. Easier said than done, right? Because once you get into your daily routine, a momentum takes over that's hard to stop. So commit right now. Pay close attention to when and why you feel hungry, how you feel while you eat, and how you feel after you eat. Take these simple steps to help you learn to listen to your body:

1. Make sure you are actually hungry before you eat. You could be bored, stressed, depressed, happy, or eating simply because there is food in front of you!

2. Eat only until you are *satisfied* today. Let's make sure we're on the same page: "satisfied" does not mean "full," "stuffed," or "sick because I ate so much"; it means you are simply *no longer hungry.*

3. Always try the water trick. Enjoy a tall glass of water before, after, or during a meal to make sure your feelings of hunger really *are* due to hunger and not thirst.

Cut the Fat

It's true there are healthy fats and unhealthy fats. Healthy fats are found in fish, nuts, avocados, olives, peanut butter, and liquid vegetable oils. Unhealthy fats are found in animal products and packaged foods. However, all fats supply a dense amount of calories—nine calories per gram of food—regardless of the "healthy" or "unhealthy" classification. And because most of us simply eat too many calories, it makes sense to cut the unnecessary fat out of your diet today.

Skip the mayo, the cream cheese, the buttered veggies, rolls, or toast, the dips, and the sauces. Try a sandwich with extra veggies, a salad with a little less dressing than usual, or a bagel with jam instead of cream cheese; by doing so you can save an average of 100 calories per serving. More important, you'll realize that the food tastes just as good and is totally acceptable without the extra fat. If you cut just *one* 100-calorie serving of fat out of your daily diet, you'll save over 36,500 calories per year! (That's about ten pounds' worth of calories.)

The Right Way to Do an Ab Crunch

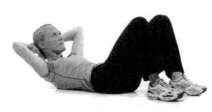

Today you can learn how to do a proper abdominal crunch. You can do these anytime—while you watch the news, with a child crawling all over you, or in your office with the door closed!

Start by lying down on the floor. Bend your knees and place your feet flat on the floor, with your toes pointing forward and your knees about shoulder width apart. Now place your hands at the base of your head, with your fingers relaxed. Keep your chin neutral—you shouldn't be pulling on your head—rather, you should be able to place a fist between your chin and your chest. Lift your head, neck, and shoulders off the floor. Squeeze your belly button in toward your spine as you lift—and as you lower! Make sure your abs are contracted both directions. If your neck feels tense, use your mental power to shift the muscular contraction to your abs.

Okay, get going. Do fifteen to twenty repetitions. Repeat two more times if you can. Exhale as you lift and inhale as you lower down. Listen to your body and take a rest whenever you need.

Relax!

It seems easy to think we'd take a moment to relax, de-stress, or enjoy a moment of peace. The reality is that most of us won't. Life is busy, and when times are tough, our mental, emotional, and/or physical needs get shoved to the bottom of our priority list.

So today make a point to do something relaxing. Your body needs a moment to de-stress—it's vital for your health and well-being.

The classic de-stress exercise is breathing—slow, controlled breathing with your eyes closed and no interruptions. Give yourself just two to five minutes to sit in a quiet area and breathe in deeply through your nose and out through your mouth. Or take a bath. Or choose to sit outside and enjoy the beauty of nature. Whatever it is, decide on a tried-and-true method of relaxation, and plan it into your busy day.

The Colorful Lunch

Quarter-pound cheeseburger: 450 calories

Large french fries: 500 calories

32-ounce soda: 300 calories

Add it all up and you get 1250 calories and 45 grams of artery-clogging fat. Yikes! Most of us need only 2000 calories and 65 grams of fat *in an entire day.*

Today, don't eat a bland lunch that consists only of dull yellow, white, or brown colors. Eat a salad for lunch—and go for color! Choose dark, leafy greens (like spinach, romaine, or endive), and top the salad with chunks of crisp veggies like carrots, cucumbers, broccoli, peas, tomatoes, or celery. Add some lean chicken, fish, or beef if you prefer, or top it with a *small* sprinkling of nuts and a sensible portion of salad dressing—about two tablespoons—on the side. Leafy greens serve as the perfect medium for mixing in a variety of healthy foods. But salads can go awry, so don't eat "taco salads" (with loads of cheese, meat, and sour cream) or add too many fatty toppings like cheese and dressing.

Avoid Activity-Zapping Traps

How often does this happen? We wait for the elevator for who-knows-how-long, when we could have easily taken the stairs in the same amount of time. We look, look, and look for the TV remote when we could have easily walked over to the television and changed the channel manually in *less* time.

Sitting quietly burns about 1.4 calories per minute.* Walking at a moderate pace burns about 5 calories per minute. Seems small, but add up the numbers time after time, day after day. Turning thirty minutes of sitting time into thirty minutes of walking time each day adds up to 39,000 calories per year—or about eleven pounds.

Great. We agree. The extra time you save isn't worth the opportunity you lose to move your muscles and burn calories! Swear off all activity-zapping conveniences today. No escalators, no elevators, no remote control. Park your car a bit farther away and enjoy the walk rather than driving around the lot looking for a better parking space (thereby spending the same amount of time in the car that you could have been walking). Be strong. I know you can do it!

---

*Figures are based on a 185-pound person.

Sticking to Your Goals: Put It on Paper

It's a futile cycle. The less you move, the less energy you have. The more you eat, the worse you feel afterward. Yet many of us still get swept away by an environment with too much food and too few opportunities to move our muscles. It's not breakthrough science: we know we have to eat healthier and exercise regularly to feel healthy and strong, yet many of us still lack the conviction to follow through with health-related goals because our environment doesn't change.

You can make that change today. Think of three reasons you want to be healthier. Do you want to have more energy? Reduce your risk for heart disease? Have the stamina to go hiking with a teenager? Maybe you want to reduce the dosage of your diabetes medicine. Or maybe you just want to feel strong and healthy. Whatever it is, write at least three reasons down. Now post your list in a visible area: on your fridge, on your desk, by the phone, or on your closet door.

The Salt Myth

I often hear people say that you shouldn't drink diet soda because it is high in sodium. The truth is that when it comes to sodium, we have other—much worse—offenders to think about. (I'm not advocating diet soda, by the way.) Take a minute to review the sodium content in commonly consumed foods:

Food	Sodium (mg)
1 serving of a packaged/boxed meal (rice, pasta, etc.)	1000
1 cup canned soup	900
1 cup cereal	90–300
1 slice white bread	225
11 potato or corn chips	180
4–5 crackers	130
1 cup milk	125
32-ounce fountain diet soda	58
12-ounce can diet soda	28
½ cup brown rice	10
1 apple	2

Try to eat no more than 2300 mg of sodium today—that's only one teaspoon of table salt. So in addition to being cautious about the sodium *in* the food you eat, be cautious about *adding* sodium—by shaking that salt shaker—to the food you eat as well.

Smart TV Time

The Bureau of Labor Statistics' 2003 American Time Use Survey found that the average American spends 2.57 hours per day watching television. Even more remarkable is the fact that 79 percent of Americans reported watching TV as a "primary activity on any given day"—second only to eating and sleeping. To top it off, national statistics show that 68 percent of us fail to get enough physical activity.

Today I recommend that you exercise while you watch TV—even if it's only for ten minutes! If you're embarrassed or need more space, send your spouse or children to another room. Do whatever you need to do. You'll burn calories, get your heart pumping, and, even better, you'll learn how easy it is to add physical activity into an already busy day.

Here are some activities that work well for TV time:

- March in place at a quick, steady pace.
- Jog in place.
- Jump rope.
- Do jumping jacks.
- Do knee lifts (raise your hands over your head, then lift your knee to about belly button height and bring your hands down and tap the knee that is lifted.)

Why Are You Eating That???

Your goal for today is to understand how your body uses calories. You don't eat just to have energy. You eat to live. You eat to feed your heart, your brain, your lungs, and every living tissue in your body. Understanding this basic principle will help you make better food choices day in and day out. If you think of food as a fuel for vital organs and tissues, common sense will begin to take over and it will become clearer what your best food choice will be.

Your body has priorities. It generally uses calories in this order:

1. Survival (heart, lungs, vital organs, etc.)
2. Comfort (hair, skin, temperature control)
3. Growth (age-related, recovery from injury, training, or disease)
4. Activity (all muscular movements, standing, running, etc.)
5. Storage (stores excess calories as fat)

Before you eat anything today, ask yourself, "Is this really *fuel* for my body? Or is it just food I want to eat to satisfy a craving?" Then try to make the best choice to fuel your vital organs and tissues.

Have a Few Spare Moments Today? Prepare Vegetables Now

If you're like me, you have a few nights a week that are all-out busy. Cooking a decent dinner on those days is not even in the scope of possibilities. On the other hand, you likely also have a few nights in which you have some time to spend in the kitchen. If tonight is one of those nights, double up your efficiency and prepare a bulk batch of vegetables so you can conveniently enjoy healthy foods for the next two to three days.

Wash and cut (if necessary) a medley of raw vegetables like carrots, broccoli, cauliflower, cucumbers, sugar snap peas, or any other favorite vegetables you have on hand. If they need to be cooked, cook the whole batch tonight.

Then divide the vegetables up into one medium-sized storage container and several individual-sized baggies. Place the containers in the fridge. The vegetables are now ready for an anytime, anywhere meal or snack. Use them for pre-meal snacks for the kids (so you don't ruin their appetites with other, not-so-healthy alternatives), in the car, or for tomorrow's dinner.

Don't Waste Your Walk

Walking is a great form of exercise because, well, we all know how to do it. You can march in place in a 2' x 2' empty space, walk outside, or really burn it up on a treadmill. But did you know the wrong form or technique while walking can actually slow you down or cause unnecessary strain to working muscles?

Go for a walk today, but make sure you use good form and technique. Here's how:

1. *Use a shorter stride.* Don't leap forward with long, lengthy strides. Rather, take short, quick steps. Land heel first; then roll through to the toes.

2. *Let your upper body lead.* Lean forward slightly from your hips and let your upper body lead the way. You want your ankles, hips, shoulders, and head in a nice, straight line—but at a slight diagonal.

3. *Keep your knees soft.* Don't let your knees lock up at any time during your walk.

4. *Pump your arms.* Bend them at a 90-degree angle, keeping the elbows in close to your body, and swing your arms back until your wrists are near your rib cage.

The Possibilities Are Endless

When a tempting treat is in sight, we often fall into a very narrow line of thinking: "To eat or not to eat the M&Ms . . . that is the question." (Poetic, I know.)

This choice is simple; choose one or the other, right? Not exactly. Be open-minded. There's a plethora of other foods from which you can choose; and there are other "productive" things you can do besides eat the M&Ms. You have the world at your fingertips. You can eat the M&Ms—or eat an apple, drink a glass of milk, eat some dried fruit, or chew some nuts. You could make a phone call, check your e-mail, read the newspaper—or do absolutely nothing.

Don't ever let yourself feel backed into a corner by a silly piece of food. Think about all your other options today. Don't ever forget how much life has to offer.

The crazy part is that sometimes it's not even about actually *wanting* the M&Ms. Sometimes it's simply about being presented with a choice: eat them or don't. And when we have those two cut-and-dried choices, the result usually involves a few M&Ms.

The Fast-Food Fix

Think simple. If you're on the run today and know you'll end up eating fast food for one of your meals, *try the dollar menu.* You'll get smaller portions, and there's no pressure to get the whole-meal deal. Don't let fast-food restaurants place extra side items in front of you that you don't really need to eat (like fries!).

Here are simple menu items you should try today to help you survive the fast-food fix:

- Small bowl of chili
- Yogurt with fruit
- Small hamburger
- Baked potato with two tablespoons sour cream
- Hamburger and yogurt
- Yogurt and chili
- Baked potato and chili
- Side salad with regular dressing
- Side salad with low-fat dressing
- Side salad and yogurt
- Side salad and chili
- Side salad and hamburger

Stand Up!

The busier we get, the more we sit. We sit at the office, we sit in the car, we sit at the movies, we sit at the computer for shopping, research, meeting, or lesson preparation—we even sit for fun.

Sitting burns about 1.4 calories per minute.* Standing burns about 3 calories per minute.

Add it up over an eight-hour time period and you get:

Sitting eight hours	686 calories
Standing eight hours	1440 calories

Wow. That's a 754-calorie difference! Try standing as much as you can today. You likely won't be able to stand for eight hours, but everything counts. And don't just stand there in a slouched position. Stand with muscular conviction and use good posture. Contract your abdominals, pull your shoulders down and back, and contract your gluteal muscles.

Stand while you talk on the phone. Stand while you watch TV. Stand during face-to-face conversations. Stand while putting gas in the car. And if you're brave, call an "all-standing" meeting.

*Figures are based on a 185-pound person.

Valentine's Day: For the Love of Chocolate

Nothing means Valentine's Day more than chocolate. Enjoy some chocolate today, but keep it under control:

- *Go for darker chocolate.* If you've heard the rumor that "chocolate is good for you," you need to know it's *dark chocolate* that actually contains more of the beneficial antioxidants (in the form of flavonoids) that are good for your heart and blood pressure. Dark chocolate is richer but is usually more satisfying, so you'll eat less chocolate overall.

- *Let it melt in your mouth.* Let the chocolate melt in your mouth so you fully taste it. If it takes you longer to eat, you'll eat less of it.

- *Spread it out over a few days.* See, I'm doing you a favor—now you get to eat chocolate for more than just one day. Really, it's better for you to not overload on a bunch of chocolate at once. You can't buy a bag or box of chocolate and expect it to "serve one." Every bag or box of chocolate will give you more than you need in a day, so eat small amounts and spread it out.

Hooked on Soda Pop?

For some of you, this may very well be one of the most difficult tasks you'll receive in this entire book.

Is all soda pop bad? In moderation, no. In excess, absolutely. If you're a regular soda drinker, "moderate" consumption would be about 12 to 24 ounces per day. "Excess" would probably equal anything over 32 ounces per day. (If you enjoy a 32-ounce—or larger—serving of soda pop once in a while, don't fret. It's those of us who must have more than 24 ounces of soda pop *every* day who need some work.) Some sodas flood your body with sugar, some with caffeine—and noncaffeinated, diet sodas (like all soda pop) simply make you miss out on drinking other healthful beverages like water, 100-percent juice, or low-fat milk.

Cut out all soda pop today. Just do it. It's only one day. You can do anything for one day! This simple exercise is beneficial—even for a day—because it helps you realize that water tastes good, too, and that you really don't *need* that soda just to get through the day. Moderation is the key.

Don't Weigh Today

Does the number on the bathroom scale affect how you feel about yourself? If you're like most Americans, it absolutely does. If the number is higher than we think it should be, many of us turn doomsday and think things like: "I'm too fat; it's hopeless to even try" or "I haven't lost any weight, so forget it!" These harsh thoughts strongly influence our actions and don't motivate us in any way to fight for our health or do positive things for our bodies.

Today, hide your bathroom scale. Feel free to keep it hidden most of the time from this point forward. It's okay to check your weight once in a while, but certainly not every day. Our bodies are all different; muscular density, bone structure, and height all affect our body weight. Think about all the great things you'll do today. You want to exercise and make wise eating choices so you can continue to do those great things. But those things likely have nothing to do with a specific number on the bathroom scale.

"I Haven't Had a Treat Since . . . "

Think about foods as either "everyday" foods or "occasional indulgence" foods. Here are some examples of each category:

Everyday Foods

- 100-percent whole-wheat bread
- Whole-grain cereal
- 100-percent whole-grain crackers or pretzels
- Fruits
- Vegetables
- Nuts/seeds/peanut butter
- Low-fat milk
- Lean meats

Occasional Foods

- Desserts
- Candy
- Salty snacks
- Ice cream
- Fast food
- Combination restaurant entrees (fettuccini Alfredo, smothered burritos, etc.)

Today, analyze what you've eaten in the last three days. Separate your food choices into the "everyday" and "occasional indulgence" categories. Write it down. How many "occasional indulgence" foods have you eaten in the past few days? (I'm guilty! I often think to myself, "Well, I can eat this today because I haven't had a treat in a long time"— when I actually forgot about the treat I ate yesterday, or right after breakfast. Oops!) This simple exercise offers a great reality check and can be repeated at any time. It's a surefire way to motivate you to do better!

10,000 Steps Today

If you already own a pedometer, set a goal to take at least 10,000 steps today.

If you don't have a pedometer, consider buying one to monitor your daily physical activity. A pedometer is a simple measuring tool that clips to your waistband and counts the number of steps you take. You can find pedometers ranging in price from $3 to $30 on amazon.com or at retail stores like Wal-Mart or Target. A pedometer is a worthy investment; it makes activity fun and motivational because you can monitor your status by the minute. You'll have a very clear picture of when you need to eat less because your day wasn't active enough, or when you need to take just a few more steps to achieve the rewarding goal of 10,000 steps per day.

Depending on your stride length, walking 1,000 steps is approximately one-half mile and 10,000 steps is approximately five miles. At a moderate three-mile-per-hour pace, 10,000 steps will burn about 500 calories.*

---

*Figures based on a 185-pound person.

5 a Day: Easier Than You Think

Twenty-two percent. That's how many Americans actually eat five servings of fruits and vegetables on an average day. Ouch.

Fruits and vegetables are packed with good nutrition, including fiber, vitamins, minerals, and phytochemicals. They are convenient, portable, and affordable. Your goal for today is to eat at least five servings of fruits and/or vegetables today. Thanks to the small portion size, it is super easy to do. Here's one way it can be done:

Breakfast: 1 serving fruit (like a banana, apple, or ½ cup berries)

Lunch: 2 servings vegetables (2 cups leafy greens topped with vegetables)

Snack: 1 serving fruit (like 1 cup cut melon, 1 pear, 1 orange)

Dinner: 1 serving vegetable (like 1 cup broccoli, carrots, or asparagus, steamed or raw)

Don't Compare

For some people it just won't sink in. Your body is amazing, miraculous, and wondrous. By simply comparing yourself to somebody else—be it looks, material possessions, or social interactions—you pile on unnecessary burdens and bring yourself down. Comparing yourself to somebody else isn't a positive experience. It isn't productive. And it doesn't motivate you to take better care of your body.

Focus on your positive attributes and learn to value the immeasurable worth of your mind, body, and spirit as they work together to create that perfect person: you! Don't ever let your day be positive or negative based on how *you* think you look. That rarely—if ever—matches what others think of us.

Don't waste time comparing yourself to anybody else today. Please.

Today, it's not about how you look. It's about how you live. So straighten up and smile. You're about to have a really good day.

Healthy Snacks on Hand

Healthy snacks can save your life. Literally. Think about the times you end up going through the drive-thru or to a restaurant to feed each member of your family a 1000 to 1500 calorie meal. Now think about it this way: what if you had had an apple and a bag of nuts in the car to tide you over until you made it home for a healthier alternative? Foods prepared at home (with healthy intention) are lower in calories, fat, sodium, and sugar—dietary culprits that can cause disease when consumed in excess.

Take thirty seconds out of your morning and pack a few healthy snacks in your purse, diaper bag, or work briefcase. This simple step can save you from overeating or from making unnecessary, unhealthy food choices. Foods like apples, oranges, pears, bananas, dried fruit, string cheese, or nuts (such as almonds or walnuts) are portable, convenient, and most of all, healthy. If healthy food is on hand, you'll have less of an excuse to cave in to the temptation of those luring, not-so-healthy alternatives.

Push-Ups Any Time, Anywhere

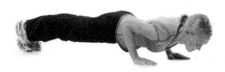

Try some push-ups today. Push-ups are a great exercise for the entire upper body and abdominals.

Set a goal to do three sets of five to twenty reps. (Just do it—you'll feel the benefits as you perform the exercise.) Here's how to do a push-up—at any fitness level:

Beginner: Get down on the floor on all fours. Move your hands out wide to the sides, in line with your shoulders; your knees should be bent directly under your hips and your abs should be contracted. Bend your elbows and lower your chest down toward the floor until your elbows are bent to a 90-degree angle. Keep your eyes looking at the floor to keep your head in proper alignment. Go down until your nose is one to three inches above the floor, then push back up.

Intermediate: Same as beginner, but walk your hands forward until your knees, hips, shoulders, and head form a straight upward diagonal line. Bring your hands in so they are directly under your chest. Keep your elbows in close to your rib cage as you lower down.

Advanced: Same as intermediate, but push up from your toes instead of your knees (see illustration).

No-Fuss Flax

Add ground flax seed to your grocery list—either for today or for your next trip to the grocery store. Ground flax seed is a very versatile health food. It tastes good and requires no special preparation. Just mix some in as you prepare your favorite dish. You can add flax seed to any muffin, cookie, pancake, waffle, bread, or casserole recipe; it even works well in hot cereal, cold cereal, or meal-replacement beverages.

You need only about one tablespoon per day to reap the benefits of flax. One tablespoon of ground flax seed has only forty calories, but it packs in two grams of fiber and 1.6 grams of the health-improving omega-3 fatty acid, alpha-linolenic acid (ALA). You don't have to eat it every day, because we do get the ALA fatty acids from other sources as well; flax seed is just one of the *best* plant sources. Flax is also packed with lignans, which are phytoestrogens; research shows lignans could possibly prevent or slow the progression of breast cancer.

Kathy Smith, Here I Come

Try a home-exercise workout video today. Dig one out of your closet or borrow one from a friend or neighbor. It could be Kathy Smith, Billy Blanks, old, new, whatever. Pick one and go for it. (Do try to pick one that was released after the year 1995 for the most accurate exercise instructions.)

If you don't have access to a home workout video, consider buying one. They can cost as little as $10 and can change your life. You don't have to have expensive equipment, you don't have to drive to a club, you don't have to dress up, and you don't have to find a baby-sitter for the kids (in fact, let them do it with you!).

Exercise will rejuvenate you and give you the energy you need to get through the day.

All Right, Who's Cooking Dinner?

My husband would find this laughable. I admit it. He doesn't come home to wife-in-apron, fine-china-on-the-table, everything's-just-perfect meals. So let's work on this one together.

Today, plan out your dinner menu for the next week. Write it down and post it in a handy location for your next trip to the grocery store (or post it in your kitchen if your pantry is already stocked). If an entire week is too overwhelming, at least figure out what you are going to prepare for dinner this evening. And don't make a mad dash to the grocery store. Some of my best meals result simply from washing and cutting (or cooking) a variety of fresh or frozen fruits and vegetables and serving them with whole-wheat cheese toast or toasted sandwiches.

Taking the time to plan ahead does work. I know from personal experience that my family eats healthier when I plan meals in advance. (It's also less expensive!) We've all been in the "what's for dinner?" mode. From there, it's all too easy to pack the kids up and go out for dinner.

Safer Meat

Read a few labels today for any meat-based products. Try to avoid eating foods with the term "mechanically separated meat" in the ingredient list. Mechanically separated meats are found in *some* hot dogs, lunch meats, chicken nuggets, sausages, and meat in boxed entrees (like frozen pizzas).

I don't want to ruin these foods for anyone, but here's a quote from Paul Brown of the National Institute of Health: "Mechanically separated meat is a paste produced by compressing carcasses, much like a used car is crushed into a dense block of metal."* That mechanical compression includes spinal cord and all. Say what?

Anyway, while this may or may not make you concerned, I hope that today you will find out what foods you have in your fridge, freezer, or shopping cart that are made with mechanically separated meats. Set a goal to eat pure chicken, turkey, pork, or beef, whenever possible, instead of their "mechanically separated" counterparts.

---

*Source: *Nutrition Action,* vol. 28, number 5, June 2001.

TIP #48

Love Hot Chocolate?

It doesn't matter whether you love to drink hot chocolate on a daily basis or only once in a while; this itsy-bitsy sacrifice will help you learn to enjoy hot chocolate in a healthier way.

Use only *one* small tablespoon of hot cocoa mix today. Or use only one-third of the powder contained in the single packets or envelopes. Why? Hot chocolate can be deceiving. One serving (2 tablespoons, or ¼ cup) of that innocent little powder can sneak twelve to twenty-eight grams of added sugar into your day. That's equal to three to seven tea-spoons of sugar, which is 30 to 70 percent of the added sugar you are allowed for an entire day—and it's in one beverage!

Trust me—you'll be surprised at how just a little cocoa mix can give plenty of flavor to a cup of warm milk. The powder will last longer, so you'll save money in the long run as well.

Just When You Need It: Time to Stretch!

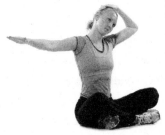

Do you ever suffer from tight back or neck muscles that cause headaches and discomfort? (I call this "lap-top syndrome"—hiked up shoulders that are rounded forward while your head presses forward toward a computer screen.)

Try this quick, relaxing stretch:

Sit up tall with your back straight, your abs contracted, and your shoulders down and back, as though you were trying to touch your shoulder blades together. Extend your right arm out to your right side. The arm should be straight and at shoulder level. Next, place your left hand on the right side of your head. Lean your head to the left and lightly press on your head with your left hand. Now, very slowly, lower your right arm down toward your right hip. You should be able to count to ten in a slow manner as you lower your arm. You'll feel the stretch as your arm nears your right hip, so take it nice and slow and give the muscles in your neck and upper back time to lengthen and relax. Repeat the stretch on the other side.

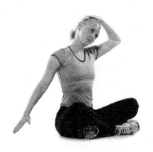

Eat Less, More Often

Set a goal to eat less than you normally do for each meal. Eat six small meals today. Think to yourself: I'm going to eat less right now, but I can eat a small snack again in just a few hours.

It's good for your body to get small, sensible portions of food at regular intervals throughout the day. You'll avoid the crazy "I'll-eat-anything" fits of starvation and you'll keep your metabolism thriving (which gives you energy and focus throughout the day). This means you get to eat four to six small meals, instead of just three square meals a day. That's good, right? See, I'm thinking of you.

Here are some simple food combinations that can be mixed and matched to equal six smaller meals:

- High-fiber cereal and milk
- Fresh fruit and string cheese
- Fresh fruit and *one* small handful of nuts
- Cottage cheese with fruit
- Peanut butter on whole-wheat bread
- Raw veggies with dip
- Tuna and celery sticks
- Light microwave popcorn and fresh fruit
- Raw veggies and nuts or cheese
- Plain or low-fat vanilla yogurt with granola or fruit

The Sweetest Dessert of All

Today is your lucky day. A dietitian is telling you to eat dessert. *Fruit* dessert, that is. Oh well, run with it.

Serve fruit for dessert tonight. These fruit desserts pack powerful doses of vitamins, antioxidants, phytochemicals, and fiber. They are also tasty, low-calorie alternatives to fat-laden sweets and desserts—great for weight loss and saving your heart and arteries from excess gunk!

- Fresh berries with low-fat yogurt or a sprinkle of sugar (or Splenda)
- Sliced peaches with low-fat milk
- Cubed cantaloupe or watermelon
- Crisp red or green grapes that have been in the freezer for two to ten minutes
- Orange slices and Craisins
- Sliced bananas and apples with fat-free Cool Whip

Dilute the Juice

Other than 100-percent orange juice, 100-percent grape juice, or 100-percent cranberry juice, I think most juices are simply too high in added sugar and calories. Really, the last thing any of us needs (especially your kids or grandkids!) is to *drink* more sugar!

Check this out:

Beverage	Sugar (tsp)
1 (20-ounce) bottle fruit juice	8–9
1 cup Sunny Delight	8
1 cup lemonade	7
1 cup apple juice	6–7
1 Capri Sun pouch	6+
1 cup Kool-Aid	4

Ideally, we shouldn't consume more than ten teaspoons per day of added sugars.

Dilute all sugary beverages today. Fill your glass with one-half juice and one-half water; or, if you're feeling brave, go with one-third juice and two-thirds water.

The Whole-Grain Hoax

Here are some common "whole-grain" claims you will see on food products in grocery stores nationwide:

- "Made with whole-wheat"
- "Good source of whole grain"
- "Multi-grain"
- "Whole-grain"
- "Now with [x] grams of whole grain!"

When you see such claims on sugary cereals, frozen pizzas, pancakes, breads, mac-n-cheese, snack/cereal bars, and even cookies, don't be fooled. It's a stretch in many cases and takes some finagling to make a "whole grain" claim on such foods. Rather than trying to understand which claim means what, here are two simple steps to help you quickly decipher whole-grain food claims:

1. Look for foods that say "100-percent whole grain." The 100 percent is the key.
2. Look at the nutrition facts label. Does the food have more than three grams of fiber? If so, it's likely a good source of whole grain.

The 2-for-1 Exercise Routine

One of the most common excuses for not exercising is "I just don't have time right now." Well, today you need to make time. Maybe if you can make it work today, you can make it work three to five days per week.

Here are some of the many ways you can combine two activities into one:

- March in place, jog, jump rope, walk on a treadmill, ride a stationary bike, or use an elliptical machine while you watch TV.
- Ride a stationary bike or use an elliptical machine while you read.
- While your kids swim at a local swimming pool, you can walk or jog laps around the pool (or a nearby area) while keeping your eye on the kids at the same time.
- While your kids play at the park, walk or jog laps around the playground.
- Walk or jog laps around your backyard while your kids play outside.
- Step up and down on the first stair of your staircase while your kids play inside or while you watch TV. You can even have a conversation with kids or a spouse while you step away.

Drowning in Maple Syrup

A nice hot meal of whole-wheat waffles, pancakes, or French toast can go from healthy to "sugar overload" in a matter of seconds thanks to maple syrup.

Compare the amount of sugar and calories in these different syrup options:

Topping	Calories	Sugar (g)	Sugar (tsp)
Homemade syrup (¼ cup)	180	44	11½
Bottled syrup (¼ cup)	200	33	8½
Jam (2 tablespoons)	112	20	5
"Sugar free" homemade syrup (¼ cup)	0	0	0

Two hundred calories may not seem like much, but remember, this is *in addition* to the waffle, pancake, French toast, butter, eggs, bacon, sausage, or whatever else you may be served with the meal.

Try making the sugar-free version of homemade maple syrup today. The recipe is simple. Combine:

2 cups boiling water
2 cups Splenda no-calorie sweetener
½ teaspoon Mapleine flavoring

This syrup tastes just as good and has *no* calories and *no* sugar. You don't want to load up on artificial sweeteners, but for a hot breakfast a few times per week, it saves so much sugar and calories, so it's definitely a good substitution.

Trans Fat: Double Trouble

Trans fats are a type of fat found in many packaged foods, restaurant foods, desserts, margarines, and shortening. They are doubly offensive to our heart health because they raise the level of LDL cholesterol (a.k.a., the "bad" cholesterol) and lower the level of HDL cholesterol (a.k.a., the "good" cholesterol).

It's interesting that people often shun stick margarine (they should), but don't think twice about eating hamburgers, decadent desserts, fried onions, or french fries, which can have anywhere from *four to eighteen* times the amount of trans fat found in stick margarine.

Read labels today and try to avoid foods with trans fat or with "partially hydrogenated vegetable oil" in the ingredient list. The average person should consume no more than twenty grams of harmful trans and/or saturated fat each day. If you will be eating meals from a restaurant, then follow these simple rules to avoid high levels of trans fat:

1. Don't order anything fried.
2. Skip appetizers (other than soup or salad).
3. Skip dessert.

Kid-Pleasing Fruits and Vegetables

Let your kids go grocery shopping with you today. It sounds like a nightmare, I know. But give it a chance.

Tell your kids that they each get to pick one fruit or vegetable of their choice. It can be something tried and true like apples, bananas, or carrots; or it can be something new to them like kiwi, tangerines, jicama, or even a fun-shaped squash. Your kids or grandkids will have fun learning about new fruits and vegetables, and they'll broaden their taste buds. Of course the big payoff is that they will be more willing to eat it—because they picked it out!

Our family trips to the grocery store are always an adventure (though not always the fun kinds!), and we've ended up with strange things like Japanese cucumbers—but my daughter at least gave the new food a try, so it was well worth it. If money is an object, tell your kids they can pick any fruit or vegetable that is under a certain price range. There is always some sort of produce in season that is affordable and nutritious.

TIP #58

There Is No Shortage of Food

I'm sure of it. At least once in my life (probably more) I had an obsession with a certain food. When presented with this food, I would eat it as fast as I could, eat more of it than I should, and hoard the rest.

One day, a simple thought crossed my mind, and it changed my relationship with food forever. It was simple: "There is no shortage of food."

I immediately realized that my favorite food would still be there tomorrow, that I could have it any time I wanted, and that there was no reason to scarf it down like a wild animal.

So are you ready? Think about that today; pace yourself when it comes to food. Learn to eat just until you are *satisfied*—not sick because you ate so much, so fast. After all, the food is not going to sprout legs and run away.

Reality Check:
Artificial Sweeteners

Artificial sweeteners are found in all kinds of foods. And even though you usually think you are consuming just *one* artificial sweetener at a time, you need to think again.

Foods like gum, diet drinks from the fountain, diet ice cream, diet cookies and candy, bottled diet fruit drinks, and even cold cereals can all offer a potential smorgasbord of artificial sweeteners such as: acsulfame K, aspartame (Nutrasweet), saccharin, sucralose (Splenda), and sugar alcohols like sorbitol, mannitol, and xylitol.

Today I hope you will simply read the ingredient list of the foods you eat—from gum to beverages to food. Find out if you are consuming more artificial sweeteners than you realize. Your goal today is to simply become *aware*. After all, some of these sweeteners *are* questionable for your health. It's always best to consume artificial sweeteners in small amounts, so try not to consume these foods in excess. So far, sucralose (or Splenda) has been proven to be a safer artificial sweetener than any of the others on the market.

New Exercise Move: Walking Lunge

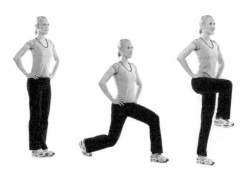

Learn how to do walking lunges today. Walking lunges are a great way to strengthen and tone your thighs, hips, and glutes.

Find an open space (your backyard, your basement, a hallway). Stand at one end of the open space so you have room to move forward. Stand with your feet about hip width apart and your toes pointing forward. Now step with your right foot forward about two feet and lower your body toward the floor until your back (left) knee is hovering two to three inches above the floor. Keep your front knee directly above the ankle—don't let the knee jet forward past your toes. Next, lift your body up and bring the left knee forward and up to hip level. Here's the walking part: now step two feet forward with the left leg and lower yourself down until the back (right) knee is hovering two to three inches above the floor. Step forward and bring the right knee up to hip level.

March in place for one to three minutes to warm up, then do two sets of ten to twenty-five reps. Listen to your body and work at your own pace. Slow and controlled is always best.

Bye Bye, White Bread

Commit to eat whole-wheat bread 100 percent of the time. Since bread is a staple part of our diet, it's vital that we make the healthiest choice possible when it comes to this everyday food. Whole-wheat bread—thanks to the nutrients found within—is protective to our health, fighting heart disease, diabetes, cancer, and obesity. Really.

Whole-wheat bread contains more fiber, protein, potassium, magnesium, vitamin E, vitamin B$_6$, copper, selenium, and zinc than its fluffy, refined counterpart. There are many versions of wheat bread out there. Look for one with three to five grams of fiber per slice and with 100-percent whole wheat indicated on the label. If you genuinely don't like wheat bread, try hard today to give it another chance. Your health is worth it. I truly believe that you can adapt your taste buds to certain foods if you believe they are good for your health.

Stress Less

We all suffer from stress at one time or another. For some of us, stress is an everyday burden. But most cases of "stressed-out-to-the-max," are caused by our own personal way of thinking. In other words, it's not always the situation that causes stress, but our own, self-conjured reaction to the situation that does.

Make a conscientious effort today not to stress over the little things. Try not to be a worrywart. Try not to stew and stress over situations that you cannot change. And try to think about one day at a time: today.

Lastly, be a positive thinker. If you're in a difficult situation, accept the reality and think about how you can move on, move forward, or improve the situation. Stewing over how difficult things are doesn't make them any easier. So don't waste your valuable time.

Need to Burn Some Calories? Try This Classic Cardio Workout

This classic pyramid cardio workout burns calories and makes time go by quickly. It can be done on a treadmill, stationary bike, or elliptical machine. It can be done on stairs or even as a basic walking workout outdoors (even at the mall). You'll be using a scale of one to ten to understand "how hard" you should be working. Here's the workout (it will take about forty minutes):

Work at This Exertion Level (on a scale of 1–10)	For This Amount of Time
2, or "very easy"	1 minute
3, or "somewhat easy"	3 minutes
4, or "moderate"	3 minutes
5, or "somewhat hard"	3 minutes
6, or "hard"	3 minutes
7, or "hard"	3 minutes
8, or "very hard"	3 minutes
9, or "very hard"	3 minutes
10, or "very, very hard"	3 minutes
8, or "very hard"	3 minutes
6, or "hard"	3 minutes
4, or "moderate"	3 minutes
3, or "somewhat easy"	3 minutes
2, or "very easy"	1 minute

Prepare Fruit in Advance

This tip works well if you've just purchased your weekly supply of fruit or if you will be buying your fruit today.

Wash and cut a medley of mixed fruit (watermelon, cantaloupe, strawberries, grapes, kiwi, mangos, or pineapple work well). Then divide the fruit into one medium-sized storage container and several individual-serving-sized baggies. Place the containers in the fridge.

The healthy fruit is now ready to go. You can pull the medium-sized bowl out and place it on the table to stave off hungry kids or spouses for pre-dinner snacking or you can grab a snack baggie on your way out the door to eat at work or in the car. How can you resist eating healthy food when it's washed, cut, and ready to go? Get all the work done at once, and then enjoy the benefits for three to five days.

"I'm Too Old to Start Exercising . . . Isn't the Damage Already Done?"

Phooey. You are *never* too old—or too young for that matter—to reap the benefits of physical activity. Exercise is critically important for good health. Your body will respond to physical activity at any age. You naturally lose muscle as you age, so you have to fight for your health more than ever as you get older. In one study, after only two months of strength training women recovered *a decade* of muscle loss and men recovered *two decades* of loss.* Not bad.

If you're concerned about your ability to participate in physical activity, get an okay from your doctor.

Here are just a few types of exercise you can try—particularly if you think you are too old to start exercising:

- Walking
- Stationary cycling
- Swimming or water walking
- Water aerobics
- Physical therapy
- Strength training (with a certified personal trainer if you are new)
- Chair aerobics (sitting in a chair and moving your feet and arms for exercise)

---

*Source: *Journal of Applied Physiology* 86 (1999): 195.

Do Carbs Really Make You Fat?

You may see this as a technicality, but it's a big one. The "wrong" kinds of carbs and large portion sizes can wreak havoc on your weight and metabolism. Carbohydrates provide essential fuel for our bodies; they are the "staff of life" when eaten in the proper form and portion size. Healthy, whole-grain carbohydrates offer up B vitamins, fiber, iron, zinc, other minerals, antioxidants, and phytochemicals that fight disease and promote good health.

Here's the breakdown on common "carb" foods and which ones you should eat more and less of:

Good Carbs: Eat More Often

- 100-percent whole-wheat bread
- Whole-grain cereal
- Whole-wheat pasta
- Brown rice
- Oats
- Vegetables
- Fruits
- Low-fat dairy foods

"Not-as-Good" Carbs: Eat Occasionally, If at All

- Soda pop
- Candy
- Chocolate
- Baked desserts
- Pastries
- Muffins
- Cinnamon rolls
- Chips
- Crackers
- Ice cream
- White rice
- White breads and rolls
- Refined pasta

Visualize the Fat

Think about fat today as greasy tablespoons of butter-flavor shortening. Got it? Good. I want you to have a clear visual image. You can even place two tablespoons of shortening in a clear plastic baggie and carry it around with you for added special effect.

Every 12 grams of fat you eat equals one tablespoon. Try to eat no more than 65 to 85 grams of fat today.

Here's the amount of fat in some common foods:

Whole milk (8 ounces)	8 grams of fat =	⅔ tablespoon
Candy bar (such as Snickers)	11 grams of fat =	about 1 tablespoon
Chicken nuggets (6 pieces)	17 grams of fat =	1½ tablespoons
Cheeseburger	21 grams of fat =	about 2 tablespoons
King-sized candy bar	22 grams of fat =	about 2 tablespoons
Salad dressing (regular, ¼ cup)	23 grams of fat =	2 tablespoons
French fries (large order)	26 grams of fat =	2 tablespoons
Grilled cheese sandwich	30 grams of fat =	2½ tablespoons
Fried chicken sandwich	30 grams of fat =	2½ tablespoons
Fettuccini Alfredo (2½ cups)	97 grams of fat =	8 tablespoons
Movie theater popcorn (large w/butter)	126 grams of fat =	10½ tablespoons
Cheese fries with ranch dressing (appetizer-sized order)	217 grams of fat =	18 tablespoons

Sources: M. F. Jacobson and J. G. Hurley, *Restaurant Confidential* (New York: Workman Publishing, 2002) and USDA Agricultural Research Service Nutrient Database for Standard Reference, Release 18.

The Work-Around-the-House Ab Workout

Think about one of those "I-really-need-to-do-that" types of projects around your house: do you almost get knocked out by junk every time you open one of your closets? Is there an area in your yard that is full of weeds? Do your windows need a good cleaning? (Sadly, the answer for me is "yes, yes, and yes!")

Pick a home-improvement project that can be reasonably carried out *today*. As you work, contract your abs tight the entire time. You'll quickly learn how beneficial it is to do two things at once.

First, make sure you know how to properly engage your abdominal muscles: contract your abdominal muscles by pulling your belly button in toward your spine. Hold the contraction and breathe two slow counts in through your nose and two slow counts out through your mouth. As you exhale, it's common to "push" your abs outward, but don't allow that to happen. Make sure your belly button stays pulled in during the exhale.

Okay, now is the time to get started. Let's face it: as the day goes on, it will be easy to say, "Forget it, I'm too busy!"

Water: Your Companion for the Day

Keep a water bottle with you at all times today. Take it with you in the car, to the office, to the kids' soccer game—everywhere.

Your body needs water to transport nutrients, remove waste and metabolic by-products, control your body temperature, protect your vital organs, and support your blood volume and circulation. Drinking water helps with weight loss as well. Your health suffers when you are dehydrated.

I'm a busy mom, and even though I know how desperately my body needs water, I sometimes get caught up in busy day-to-day life and forget to drink water. But the days I tote around a twelve- to twenty-ounce water bottle, I stay on top of my water needs with very little effort.

You can drink too much, so don't go too overboard with this. Most women need about 90 ounces per day and most men need about 125 ounces per day. You'll get about 20 percent of that need through solid food. And keep in mind that high temperatures, humidity, and exercise can increase your water needs.

Enjoy the Foods You Love ... Healthfully

Half. That's your rule for the day.

All foods can fit into a balanced diet, and if you love chocolate cake, fettuccini Alfredo, or pizza, then great, enjoy it today. Just make sure you *promise yourself* that you are going to eat only one-half of what you are served or one-half the amount you usually consume. Share the entrée with your spouse, your child, a friend, a coworker, or simply take the other half home for the next day. If eating less leaves you starving for something more, fill the void with fruits, vegetables, or a small handful of nuts.

The purpose of this? To help you train your mind and your appetite to be satisfied with less. This is something all of us—young, old, fit, unfit, active, sedentary, whatever—need to learn. Our bodies have become adapted to gigantic portion sizes that are simply uncalled for. It's going to take some serious effort to retrain ourselves to appreciate delicious food served in smaller portions.

Short on Time? Then Shorten Your Workout

Busy day today? No problem. You can shorten your workout by up to half if you simply work out at a higher intensity. Check this out:

Activity	Speed	Duration	Calories Burned*
Walking	3 mph (moderate)	30 minutes	150
Running	6 mph (fast)	30 minutes	428
Cycling	10 mph (leisurely)	30 minutes	170
Cycling	14–16 mph (fast)	30 minutes	430

See the difference? Fifteen minutes of working out at a higher intensity burns more calories than working for twice as long at the lower intensity!

Still, you should always listen to your body. It's perfectly okay to slow down for thirty to ninety seconds in the middle of an intense workout in order to give your muscles (or your breathing) a break. Just pick back up when you are ready. Make sure you can speak and breathe in a controlled manner to ensure you are working at a safe, effective level. If you can't speak during the workout, you're working too hard.

If you have a possible medical condition that would prohibit you from working at a more intense level, talk with your physician before changing your exercise routine.

---

*Figures based on a 185-pound person.

Does Lack of Sleep Cause Weight Gain?

The research isn't 100-percent conclusive, but recent studies lead us to believe that our sleep habits do affect our weight in the following ways:

1. Sleeping less means you're awake more; this means you tend to eat more—and often in the late evening, which is even worse.
2. Research studies have shown that sleeping less causes a change in the hormones leptin and ghrelin.* Leptin tells your body to *stop* eating. Ghrelin tells your body to *keep* eating. When you sleep less, your brain sends signals that drop leptin levels, lower metabolic rate, and boost your hunger level. This scenario puts you at risk for weight gain—and that's without eating any extra food. Yikes! Maybe it's time to stop *intentionally* depriving ourselves of valuable sleep time.

Research conducted at Columbia University* found the following:

6 hours sleep = 23% more likely to be obese than those who slept 7 to 9 hours
5 hours sleep = 50% more likely to be obese
4 hours sleep = 73% more likely to be obese

The research is compelling. I hope it gives you the conviction you need to get 7 to 8 hours of sleep tonight. Make it a priority.

---

*Source: David Schardt, Nutrition Action, vol. 32, no. 6, July 2005 (Center for Science in the Public Interest).

Old-Fashioned Oatmeal

Compare oatmeal to a few other cereals:

1-Cup Serving	Calories	Fiber (g)	Sugar (g)	Sodium (mg)
Cheerios	110	3.5	1	213
Flavored instant oatmeal	157	2.8	12.5	253
Frosted Mini-Wheats	175	5	10	5
Lucky Charms	114	1.5	13	203
Old-fashioned rolled oats	147	4	.5	2
Raisin Bran	187	7.1	16.5	289

Eat one cup (cooked) of good old-fashioned rolled oats today—not the microwavable instant packets—but plain oats without added sugar. Oats are high in fiber, low in sugar, low in salt, and very filling. Oatmeal even packs as much protein as a glass of milk or an ounce of meat. One small bowl can calm your appetite for hours. You can add one-fourth cup of fresh berries or a teaspoon of brown sugar (which adds a meager fifteen calories).

Oatmeal is perfect for meals *and* snacks. And let's not forget the best part: You can prepare a meal in two minutes.

Spiritual Motivation

Most of us know what steps we *should* take to improve our health. Eat more fruits and veggies. Drink more water. Eat less fat. Eat less everything. Exercise more. Does any of this sound like breakthrough science? Likely no. We've heard all this before—so why is it so hard to follow through with these basic health principles? Life is busy; that's for sure. Sometimes you just don't have the time or the resources to make the healthiest choice. But let's be honest—sometimes we simply lack the motivation to make better choices.

If you suffer from lack of motivation today, read Doctrine and Covenants section 89. It's only twenty-one verses long, and it teaches and reminds us about our great "principle with promise": the Word of Wisdom. The Word of Wisdom clearly tells what we should eat in order to be spiritually and physically strong—helping us to feel our best and live to our full potential. Verses 18 to 21 explain the benefits of obeying the Word of Wisdom; those verses are especially inspirational, encouraging, and motivational.

The Best Bedtime Snack

Fresh fruit and a glass of low-fat milk or a small handful of almonds or walnuts.

That's the best snack before bed. (See, I'm thinking of you. I just got right to the point.)

Hands down, this is a healthy, convenient snack that's perfect for bedtime. The fruit will calm a craving for sweets and provide a good dose of vitamins and fiber. Other common snacks are too high in calories, fat, sugar, and/or sodium. For example:

Ice cream: 1 small cup has 300 calories, 1 tablespoon of fat, and over 8 teaspoons of sugar.

Butter-flavor microwave popcorn: 1 small *snack* bag has 250 calories, 1½ tablespoons of fat, and 300 mg of sodium.

Cookies and milk: 2 cookies with 1 cup of milk contains 400 calories, 8 teaspoons of sugar, and 1½ tablespoons of fat.

Chips and soda pop: 2 ounces of chips and a 12-ounce can of soda pop contain 450 calories, 1½ tablespoons of fat, and 600 mg of sodium (that's about half the sodium you should have in an entire day).

These days, snacks are so hefty, they are like a meal. Choose wisely.

"I Shouldn't Have Eaten So Much!"

If you've eaten too much lately, skip breakfast today to make up for it. If you ate too much today, skip breakfast tomorrow to make up for it.

Drink a glass of water for breakfast and then eat a healthy lunch and dinner to balance your unhealthy day with a healthier day. Skipping meals *once in a while* is acceptable. But try not to intentionally skip meals more than once a week. Starving yourself on a regular basis confuses your body, leading to fat storage and muscle wasting—two things that can really slow your metabolism. And it's a long road back to get that metabolism revved back up. (The only way you can really increase your metabolism is through regular strength training and consistently eating small meals throughout the day.)

Balancing out your calorie intake—eating less food after a period of eating too much food—is an essential part of learning to listen to your body, learning to accept your body, and learning to have a positive relationship with food.

The Diversion Trick: Kids and Healthy Foods

If your children or grandchildren refuse to eat certain health foods, introduce the food during TV time or play time. Sneak a plate of sliced fruit or vegetables or a 100-percent whole-wheat bread sandwich in front of them while they are distracted. You know, while they are watching a favorite movie, playing a favorite game, or reading their favorite books or stories.

I'm continually surprised at the stuff I see kids eat when they are busy with another activity. Wheat bread, steamed broccoli, kiwi, and all sorts of different foods have been introduced in homes with no squawking, no complaining, and no "eeeeews" thanks to good old-fashioned diversion. Sure, you want to eat most of your meals at the table, but this is an effective here-and-there sacrifice that is only short term. Your children are developing their taste likes and dislikes right now. (No pressure.) So it is important for you to continue to introduce healthy foods so that kids—ages one to eighteen—can learn to tolerate and enjoy healthy foods. It can take up to ten introductions before a child will actually accept a new food. So don't give up easily.

Do It for Your Cholesterol

High blood pressure has been called "the silent killer"—people don't realize they have it, but it can end a life without much notice. High cholesterol works the same way; it doesn't always cause pain; you can't feel it. But it can lead to disease or premature death. So if no form of motivation has worked for you yet, do it for your cholesterol! And *so what* if you have perfectly controlled cholesterol? That's no guarantee that you won't have to worry about it later.

Your blood cholesterol can be elevated due to:

- Eating too much saturated fat
- Eating too many trans fats
- Not exercising on most days of the week
- Genetics

Today, put up a fight to improve and/or maintain healthy blood cholesterol levels.

Do one of these things to improve or maintain cholesterol:

- Eat more fiber, fresh fruits, and vegetables.
- Replace the bad fats (saturated and trans) with good fats (plant fats like canola or olive oil, nuts, seeds, avocados, or fish oils).
- Exercise, including strength training, on most days of the week.

Label Watch

Read the nutrition facts label for everything you eat today. Don't worry—you don't have to memorize the calories of everything you eat. You don't even have to be looking for anything in particular. You simply need to become aware of what you put into your mouth. Check out your favorite foods in your cupboards, or take ten seconds to review the labels of only the foods you actually eat today. It's kind of like building a mental filing system in your head: you remember things like "well, the fat-free cookies had 130 calories per serving" and "the regular cookies had 110 calories per serving." Hmmm.

Here are some significant things you can review on a nutrition label:

- Servings per container (watch for tricky ones like soda pop: 2.5 servings per container—but who only drinks 40 percent of a bottle of soda?)
- Serving size (watch out—it's usually small)
- Calories (don't eat too many . . .)
- Fat (eat *less*)
- Sugar (eat *less*)
- Sodium (eat *less*)
- Fiber (eat *more*)

The Best Veggie Dip

If you have a hard time truly enjoying the taste and texture of certain vegetables, or, if it's a "task" to eat your vegetables and you don't enjoy them, try dipping the vegetables in salsa. Salsa complements the flavor of many vegetables, and it has a lot less calories and fat than creamy dips or cheese sauces.

Here's the lowdown on the "veggie dips":

¼-Cup Serving	Calories	Fat (g)
Ranch salad dressing	280	28
Ranch dip (made with sour cream)	140	10
Ranch dip (made with fat-free sour cream)	116	1.6
Cheese (sauce or grated)	118	9
Salsa	17	0

Salsa is the best choice for veggie dipping, hands down. Try some today!

New Exercise Move: Triceps Dip

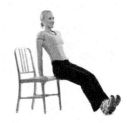

Triceps dips strengthen and tone the back of your arms, along with your shoulders and abdominals (which help stabilize the movement).

Here's how to do proper triceps dips with a chair:

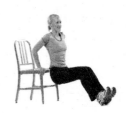

Sit on a sturdy chair, a bench, or a bottom stair. Place your hands on the chair at your sides with palms downward and fingers pointing toward your knees. Step your feet one to two feet in front of you, and then raise your buttocks off the chair. Bring your hips forward (toward your toes) about two inches. Keep your shoulders above your wrists. Now lower yourself down two to six inches until your shoulders are in line with (or just above) the elbows. Push back up to the starting position. Keep your abs contracted as you lift and lower.

Warm up by marching in place and really pumping your arms for one to three minutes. Try to do one to three sets of ten to twenty repetitions. Listen to your body; it's okay to do more or less.

The Good Things about You

Think about this: focusing on the things we don't like about ourselves doesn't make us feel any better. And it doesn't help us make long-term changes that are maintainable and realistic. It just makes us feel bad. And yet many of us waste valuable time and energy each and every day with such negative, nonproductive thoughts.

Focus on these things instead:

- The things you like about you.
- The people you like to be with and who like to be with you.
- The things that make you happy.

Good. Now write your thoughts down on paper. Try to come up with at least two positive things in each area. Keep these thoughts on your mind today. If a negative thought about you pops into your head at some point, try to quickly change your thoughts to the positive things you took note of earlier.

Focusing on "the good things about you" gives you the priceless motivation, self-confidence, and self-conviction to take better care of your body.

TIP #83

Simple Ways to Reduce Stress

It's funny. I'm about to tell you to *add* something to your day in order to *reduce* your stress level. Well, not really. Let me explain:

Drop at least one *unnecessary* daily activity (like watching TV); in exchange, find five to thirty minutes of peaceful meditation to get your mind and priorities in order. Try one of these today:

- Do five to thirty minutes of exercise (cardio or strength activities like walking, cycling, stair stepping, weight lifting, etc.).
- Try deep, controlled breathing: close your eyes and inhale slowly for four seconds then exhale slowly for four seconds. Try to do at least eight sets of controlled breathing (four-second inhale and four-second exhale).
- Do five to ten minutes of light stretching.
- Do five minutes of meditation. (What are your goals for the day *and today only?* Think about one day at a time.)
- Listen to inspirational music for five to thirty minutes.
- Think positively for at least five minutes. (If you're in a tough situation, accept it as a reality and think about how you can improve the situation or simply move forward.)

The Popcorn You Should Eat

I once read a nutrition book that exposed the calories, fat, and sugar content of common movie theater snacks. The book, titled *Restaurant Confidential,* labeled movie theater snacks as a "Horror Show."

It used to be that you could eat high-fat popcorn only at the movie theater, but that is no longer the case. High-fat popcorn is now all over the supermarket shelves and sitting right in our own cupboards. It's just, well, scary.

Today, try eating *plain* popcorn for a snack. It's a good source of fiber and it's filling. Think plain popcorn is too bland? Review the popcorn comparison chart below. Plain popcorn might taste a bit better when you see how much healthier it is for you.

6-Cup Serving*	Calories	Fat (g)
Plain microwave popcorn	180	2
Microwave "butter flavor" popcorn	250	17
Movie popcorn popped in vegetable shortening	310	19
Movie popcorn with "butter"	540	32

---

*Six cups is a commonly consumed individual serving size. Three cups is the recommended serving size. A "large" movie theater popcorn container holds 20 to 30 cups!

Calcium Check: Are You Getting Enough?

Male, female, young, old—we all need calcium for vital reasons, yet none of us seem to get enough of it.

Write down everything you ate yesterday. Slowly think about each meal and snack one at a time—and in detail.

Okay, check your list and circle any of the following foods:

- Milk (1-cup serving)
- Cheese (1-ounce serving)
- Yogurt (1-cup serving)
- Tofu (½-cup serving)
- Calcium-fortified orange juice or cereal with 25 percent of the Daily Value or DV (1-cup serving)

Now count 300 mg of calcium *per serving* for every circled food on your list. (If you had a 16-ounce glass of milk, for example, that adds up to 600 mg.)

Next, add an extra 300 mg to account for the miscellaneous sources of calcium in your diet (like leafy greens, green vegetables, beans). Now total the numbers. How'd you do? This is not exact, but gives you a general idea. If you're aged eighteen to fifty-five, you should try to consume 1200 mg of calcium per day. Those aged fifty-five and older should strive for 1500 mg per day.

Easter: How to Survive the Candy Parade

It feels like it's raining candy every time Easter rolls around—it's like the spring version of Halloween. Kids get candy from too many places: Easter egg hunts, parents, grandparents, even school. Then all that candy sits around the house for days or weeks and tempts everyone to indulge a little—or a lot—every day.

This year, try to tone down the candy focus:

- If grandparents or other family members typically give your kids candy, then *don't* you give the kids any more. Instead give them hard-boiled eggs, a book about Easter, a spring coloring book, or sunglasses, and so forth.
- Pick *one* Easter egg hunt to attend this year.
- Don't put the candy in candy dishes. Keep it in the cupboard and keep bowls of fruits or wheat crackers out in sight.
- If you want to share the sugar at the office, don't put out a huge, never-ending candy dish. Put out a moderate amount of candy (so coworkers get one serving) and then put the dish away until the next day.
- Focus on the real meaning of Easter and Jesus Christ.

"Thinner People Are Not Happier"

If you're a woman, chances are you've thought the unthinkable at least once in your life: "If I could lose just ten pounds I'd be happier," or "I bet so-and-so is happier than me; she doesn't have to worry about her weight," or maybe, "She eats anything she wants and never gains a pound! It's not fair!"

On paper, such logic looks ridiculous. The presumption that "thin" people are "happier" is just plain silly, right? But in real life, these are real thoughts that come into our minds—and we have to deal with them.

Today, I want you to realize that such presumptions are simply untrue. Worse, they only create negative feelings about yourself and others. *Everyone* has trials and problems. While some may struggle with weight, others may struggle with different trials that are just as heart wrenching. All you can do is work on you. Exercise, eat the best you can, and work on your attitude. A positive attitude is what makes you vibrant, healthy, and happy—on the inside and on the outside.

TIP #88

The Secret to Healthy Snacking

Eat your snack foods (like chips, pretzels, dry cereal, candy, crackers, etc.) on a plate. Take *one* handful or one serving and place it on the plate. Then seal the container or bag tightly and put it away—in the cupboard and out of sight!

If you can't see the food, it won't be as tempting to keep eating extra servings or to mindlessly eat handful after handful. You know, like those times when you think "I'll just eat a few crackers" and before you know it half the box is gone. Even worse, if you eat it mindlessly, you didn't taste it or enjoy it! What a shame. (I know from personal experience.) Studies have shown that having large amounts of food placed in front of you means one thing: you eat more—much more—than you would have if you had been given a smaller serving size.

Healthier Food Gifts and Service Projects

Nothing says "thank you" or "get better" like a plate of sweet sugar and artery-clogging fat. That's what most of us give when we make plates of cookies, brownies, sweet breads, or cake. Gee, thanks!

Don't worry—I'm not really that cold-hearted. You can still make sweet treats for those you care about. In fact, I love to receive those goody plates just as much as the next person.

But today, try making a "healthy" plate for that neighbor, family member, or coworker in need. Thank those close to you with something that will help them feel good in the long run. (Sugar and fat do taste great, but it's only a short-term feeling.)

In an ideal world, we'll eventually learn to "balance" those treat plates. Sometimes we will give the gift of chocolate and tasty treats. Sometimes we will give the gift of health *and convenience:* like a plate of washed, cut, and ready-to-eat fruit and/or vegetables or a loaf of home-made whole-wheat bread.

Mystery Vegetables

Are you in a rut? Do you prepare the same array of vegetables week in and week out? Different vegetables have different qualities, so eating a variety of veggies is good for your health, giving you more nutrients and broadening your taste buds to enable you to enjoy new healthy foods.

Try a new vegetable you've never tried before. For example:

- Arugula
- Bok choy
- Sweet potatoes
- Cassava (cooked)
- Chard
- Jicama
- Kale
- Okra

There are many more uncommon vegetables from which to choose. Take a minute to wander in the produce section of the grocery store. Many stores offer little cards with cooking tips and recipe ideas right next to the vegetables. If you aren't sure how to prepare, eat, or cook a certain vegetable, do a quick search at www.about.com on the vegetable of your choice.

Great-Tasting Granola

Try this delicious homemade granola recipe. It's easy—I promise! You can serve a one-half cup serving of this scrumptious granola in yogurt, with fresh fruit, or as a cold cereal, or you can mix it with nuts and dried fruit for your own trail mix. This granola is high in healthy mono-unsaturated fat, fiber, and protein. It's good for you, but also calorie dense—so eat small, one-half cup servings.

Homemade Granola

8 cups old-fashioned rolled oats
1 cup brown sugar
1 cup wheat germ
½ cup canola or olive oil
1 cup cold water
1 tablespoon vanilla
1 teaspoon salt
Cinnamon for sprinkling

Preheat the oven to 250 degrees. Mix the oil, water, vanilla, and salt together in a large bowl. Then add the oats, brown sugar, and wheat germ and mix thoroughly. Cover a large baking sheet with aluminum foil. Pour the mixture onto the baking sheet and sprinkle with cinnamon (optional). Bake for 50 minutes if you like it softer or 60 minutes if you like it crunchier. Stir the mixture after 30 minutes.

Nutrients per ½-cup serving: 270 calories, 11 grams fat (1.5 grams saturated), 8 grams protein, 5 grams fiber.

Commit to Get Fit

This is not a "today-only" goal. This tip is actually something you need to *commit to* today, but follow through with for the next seven days.

Set a goal for the week: you need to exercise for thirty minutes at least five of the seven days this week. One week. That's all. Don't be overwhelmed; just try it. If you already work out every day, simply commit to continue down this beneficial path.

Exercise is beneficial for every muscle, every tissue, and every cell in your body. It improves blood flow and nutrient delivery, boosts metabolism, and helps your heart and lungs to be stronger and more efficient (meaning they don't have to work so hard day after day). You don't do this just to "get thinner"—it's something you need to do to ward off disease and to feel your best! We have to make time for physical activity. Sure, life is busier than ever, and you'll have good and bad weeks—sometimes working out six days and sometimes working out only one day. But always keep it a daily priority. The quality of your life depends on it.

TIP #93

Three Servings of Fruit

Choose to eat at least three servings of fruit today. Choose from apples, bananas, oranges, pears, peaches, tangerines, apricots, cherries, cantaloupes, watermelons, honeydews, plums, kiwis, mangos, papayas, pineapples, grapes, pomegranates, strawberries, raspberries, blueberries, and any of the other berries. And those are just the "normal" fruits. There are many more from which you can choose.

One serving equals:

- 1 whole medium-sized fresh fruit
- 1 cup sliced or cubed fresh fruit
- ½ cup berries
- ¼ cup dried fruit

Fruits are now increasingly available year round, so take advantage and enjoy the refreshing good taste of wholesome fruit as much as you can.

(Sometimes we hesitate to pay $4 for a cantaloupe during the winter, but then we buy snack foods for the same price without thinking twice. We get a little trapped by the "it's too expensive" mind-set simply because a fruit is not in season; but try comparing the price of fruit to other snack foods you are willing to spend money on year-round. Is it possible to make a swap with your food dollars?)

Live Guilt-Free Today

You know the routine: you feel guilty for not exercising better so you stop exercising all together. Or maybe you feel guilty for having an over-the-top dinner, so you say "I already blew it" and top it off with dessert. Guilt is our worst enemy when it comes to our health habits. Feeling guilty about our food choices, exercise habits, and our presumed defective weight or shape isn't beneficial for any of us. Guilt leads to "all-or-none" thinking: "I already messed up, so why try? I give up!" Just don't go there.

Guilt-free health thoughts are like "moving on"; they help you build a healthy relationship with food and exercise. Guilt-free thoughts take away the punishment mind-set and give you the power to take initiative to *counterbalance* those not-so-healthy choices. For example: "I ate a piece of cake, so I'm going to walk on the treadmill for thirty minutes tonight" or "I couldn't resist those warm cookies, so I'm going to eat a fresh salad for dinner."

Stuck in a Hotel? Try This 25-Minute Workout

This is a cardio workout that can be done in any hotel room with a 5' x 5' square space. Play some fast music if possible—about 130 to 140 beats per minute. The music will really motivate you to keep a steady pace.

March in place
(with high knees!)

Step touch
(wide arms!)

Hamstring curls
(reach back with arms)

Squat side to side
(like sitting in a chair)

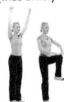
Knee lifts
(tap knee with hands)

1st Circuit: Perform each move for 1 minute at a slow, warm-up pace.

2nd Circuit: Perform each move for 1 minute at a moderate pace.

3rd Circuit: Perform each move for 1 minute at a vigorous pace.

4th Circuit: Perform each move for 1 minute at a moderate pace.

5th Circuit: Perform each move for 1 minute at a slow, cool-down pace.

Eat What You Want . . . Just Eat Less of It!

Pledge to follow this simple rule today:

Eat what you want—but only *one* serving of each food for the entire day.

So if you want some M&Ms, you are allowed one-fourth of a cup (measure it, or eat one small handful). Then that's it. You're done with M&Ms for today. If you want to enjoy a regular, high-sugar, high-calorie soda pop, you get eight ounces today. That's one serving and only 40 percent of a twenty-ounce bottle. Be strong. You can do it. It's only one short day!

The idea is to train yourself to know, understand, and be satisfied with one serving. It won't happen in a day, but this will be a good start. Oftentimes, trying something once is an unforgettable experience. You may fall off the wagon here and there and go back to your old ways, but the healthier way of eating "one serving at a time" will always pop back into your mind as a method for helping you look and feel your best.

The 10 Best Snacks Found in a Gas Station

If you are on the road today, or if your day is so busy that you are forced to grab some attempted nourishment from a gas station, try one of these healthy alternatives. You'll avoid sabotaging your health as you leave the high-sugar, high-fat, high-calorie contenders where they belong: on the shelf. And you'll feel better for it.

Here are ten healthy choices available in most gas stations or convenience stores:

1. Bottled water
2. Low-fat milk
3. Yogurt (light, low-fat, or plain)
4. Nuts (don't eat the whole bag, have one to two handfuls only)
5. Energy bars such as Clif, Pria, Nutri-grain, or Kashi
6. String cheese
7. Sunflower seeds
8. Fig Newtons
9. Toast and peanut butter crackers
10. Beef jerky (with 600 mg of sodium, make sure you eat *one* serving)

Even the healthy alternatives can be problematic if you consume too much. So watch the serving sizes.

Grocery Store Smarts: Healthy Grocery Shopping

"Fresh is best." This rule is simple but immensely beneficial. At the grocery store, shop for foods from the "outer" aisles of the grocery store. Stick to fruits, vegetables, low-fat dairy, lean meats, and 100-percent whole-grain breads. You can venture into the middle aisle for a box or two of whole-grain cereal (I love the Kashi brands and old-fashioned oatmeal), a box of instant brown rice, a few cans of beans, and maybe a package of whole-wheat pasta. Try to spend at least 80 percent of your grocery dollars on the outer, "fresh food" aisles.

Once you get the fresh foods home, make them a priority. Eat them before you eat canned, frozen, or packaged foods. Fresh foods will spoil, and you may end up wasting your money if you put off eating the healthy foods first. Try to avoid the "I'll just cook some frozen peas and steam that broccoli tomorrow night" syndrome. That cycle can continue all week—until the wholesome foods end up in the garbage.

TIP #99

Sweeten Sour Fruit

One day I was eating a bowl of fresh strawberries. They were a little sour, so I sprinkled some sugar on them. My friend looked at me and said, "I don't like strawberries . . . and I can't believe you are adding sugar to them. Doesn't that defeat the purpose?" She may have had a good point until she unwrapped a candy bar and ate that instead.

Two cups of sliced strawberries have a full day's supply of vitamin C, along with folate, potassium, and fiber. A typical candy bar has 28 grams of sugar, 250 calories, and 10 to 15 grams of fat.

If you ever have to choose between eating some fruit with a little sugar sprinkled on top or a sweet snack (like candy bars, cookies, other sweet foods), definitely choose the fruit!

If there is a type of fruit you don't eat because you don't like the taste, try it today, with a teaspoon of sugar to sweeten the deal. For zero calories and zero grams of sugar, you can try an artificial sweetener such as Splenda or sucralose.

The Best Exercise Program for Weight Loss

The best program for weight loss includes strength training two to three days per week and interval cardio training three to five days per week.

Strength training makes you strong, lean, and healthy. It builds strong bones and fights osteoporosis. It creates life-pumping, energy-infused muscles that burn more calories and fat, thus increasing your metabolic rate.

Interval cardio training means you alternate periods of higher intensity exercise with periods of lower intensity exercise. On a scale of one to ten, with one being little or no effort and ten being maximum effort, you might bounce from a level three to an eight and back to a three and so on. The higher intensity should feel "challenging," but you should still be able to speak. The lower intensity should feel "comfortable."

Today, write down your exercise program for this week; what are you going to do on each day of the week? If strength training is on your agenda, allow a day of rest between each strength training day.

Note: Start things off right by consulting with a personal trainer, or spend a few dollars on hand weights or resistance tubing that come with how-to workout instructions.

TIP #101

The Encourage-You-to-Snack-Healthy Table Centerpiece

Find a nice basket or bowl for your table centerpiece. Fill it full of some kind of fruit like apples, pears, oranges, bananas, mangos, papayas, or kiwis. You can even put a loaf of whole-wheat bread—package and all—in the basket, along with a few whole-wheat pretzels or crackers. A few colorful vegetables like cucumbers, peppers, or squash will top it off beautifully. If you are worried about spoilage, purchase a small centerpiece basket, or don't fill the basket too full. Just put enough in there to eat for the day and replenish the basket every morning. And if the only thing you have in your kitchen—right now, on this surely busy day—is a couple of apples, then great, put two apples in a basket on your table and call it good. Making *any* healthy food visible in your kitchen will be advantageous.

Having healthy food not only in front of you but arranged in an eye-pleasing basket or bowl will inspire you and your family to first eat something healthy.

Be Reasonable

If you feel yourself being tempted by the latest "lose ten pounds in the first week!" rapid weight-loss gimmick, ponder this thought: do you know *anybody* for whom a rapid weight loss program has actually worked—permanently? Losing weight rapidly (more than three pounds a week) involves restricting and depriving yourself of things you need, enjoy, and love. It never lasts, and it usually ends with a complete meltdown—creating or perpetuating an unfortunately unhealthy relationship with food.

The reality is hard to accept: there is no magic potion. Losing weight is hard work. There are no good or bad foods, but there are *limits* and *guidelines* to help you learn how to enjoy all foods in a sensible, practical, and moderate way.

Set a reasonable goal: try to eat less junk, eat more fruits and vegetables, and be more physically active. By doing so, you can lose one to two pounds per week, which is realistic, totally doable, and much, much more healthy for you in the long run.

If you want to be healthy for a lifetime, you have to work on it for a lifetime. Period.

The Best Snacks for the Road

If you're like any American, chances are you'll spend some portion of your day riding in a car. Take advantage of this time to eat something healthy. This will help you avoid a fast-food run, a gas-station junk-food raid, or even skipping meals altogether (which is not healthy for your metabolism).

Put at least one of these snacks in your car today:

- Apples
- Pears
- Bananas
- Baby carrots
- String cheese
- Nuts
- Dried fruit
- Whole-wheat crackers or pretzels
- Bottled water
- Dry cereal (a high-fiber kind with more than three grams of fiber per serving)
- Seeds (like sunflower or pumpkin)
- Plain popcorn
- Plain granola bars

Some of these foods (like cereal, nuts, bottled water, crackers, etc.) can stay in your car for several days to a week or more, depending on your climate. So all you have to do is put the stuff in your car today and enjoy the convenience of ready-to-go snacks in your car all week.

A New Power Food: Beans

Eat some beans today. Try black beans, pinto beans, garbanzo beans, or kidney beans. If you're a fabulous cook or have time to spend in the kitchen, go ahead and cook your own beans. But if you're busy and looking for fast and healthy fixes, use canned beans. Rinse the beans and mix them into a dinner entrée or a fresh salad. Try eating them plain as a main dish. You can also try one-half cup of beans wrapped in a whole-wheat tortilla with some salsa.

Beans are not fully recognized as the powerful health food they deserve to be. They are a wonderful source of protein, fiber, and carbohydrates (which provide essential fuel for your brain and muscle tissue). Because they are a plant food, they're also a source of phytochemicals: nutrients that fight and protect our bodies against common diseases. After enjoying a serving of beans today, try to eat beans two to three times per week, if possible.

The Must-Try 30-Minute Strength Workout—No Equipment Necessary!

This workout is all about efficiency, convenience, and yes, good old-fashioned hard work. It takes as little as thirty minutes and can help keep your heart healthy, your metabolism revving, your mind at peace, and your body full of vitality and strength through these very busy times.

Try this thirty-minute strength training workout today:

1. Basic squat: 15 reps (see Tip #10)
2. Push-ups: 15 reps (see Tip #43)
3. Triceps dips: 15 reps (see Tip #81)
4. Walking lunge: 15 reps (see Tip #60)
5. Ab crunch: 25 reps (see Tip #22)

Rest one to two minutes and repeat sequence. Then march in place or walk around for three to five minutes to cool down.

Confused about Vitamin Supplements? You're Not Alone

None of us eats perfectly, so it's a good idea to take a basic multivitamin to protect our health. Check yours today to see if it matches these two main guidelines:

1. *Approximately 100 percent of the Daily Value for most of the nutrients.* Watch out for too much; don't be deceived by the "more is better" mind-set. Also, it's *okay* to have less than 100 percent of the DV for the following*:

   - *Calcium.* Take calcium as a separate supplement (or make sure you consume three servings per day of milk, cheese, or yogurt).
   - *Vitamin E.* New research has shown that high doses of vitamin E can actually be detrimental to your health.
   - *Vitamin A (actetate or palmitate).* Too much can increase the risk of hip fractures. Ideally, you should look for a multiple vitamin with no more than 60 percent of the Daily Value—because you get vitamin A from food as well.

2. *The symbol: "USP" for United States Pharmacopeia.* This doesn't automatically mean the supplement is *safe.* But it does mean the ingredients in the supplement will actually dissolve.

---

*Source: Bonnie Liebman and David Schardt, *Nutrition Action,* vol. 33, no. 2, March 2006 (Center for Science in the Public Interest).

Laughter:
The Best Medicine

Enjoy a good laugh today. Not just because it makes you happy, but because it can help you deal with stress—something mentally and physically taxing. A good laugh can improve your blood pressure, reduce stress hormones and muscle tension, improve your overall sense of well-being, and bring you into an instant state of relaxation.

Here are a few ways to help you find a good laugh today:

- If you are in a stressful situation, visualize yourself in a funny circumstance instead.
- Laugh at yourself. (One day I headed to a city ninety miles away from my home. When I arrived, I realized I had no money, no wallet, and only one-eighth of a tank of gas! Oops. The only way I got through it was to laugh at myself. Pretty soon, my friends were offering me money and it wasn't the least bit embarrassing. In fact, it provided a great laugh for all involved, which was an instant stress reliever.)
- Surround yourself with bright, happy people who can help you see the humor that surrounds you every day. (Kids are great at this.)

What Is a "Healthy" Weight?

Life shouldn't ever be about how much you weigh. And judging your personal health status should never depend solely on your weight. Your body weight is just one part of the picture. Your percent body fat and your body mass index, what you eat 80 percent of the time, and how much you exercise are all equally important in assessing your level of health (and risk of disease).

Take a moment to estimate your healthiest body weight.

For Women

1. Start with 100 pounds for five feet.
2. Add five pounds per inch over five feet.
3. Subtract 10 percent for a small body frame.
4. Add 10 percent for a large body frame.

For Men

1. Start with 106 pounds for five feet.
2. Add six pounds per inch over five feet.
3. Subtract 10 percent for a small body frame.
4. Add 10 percent for a large body frame.

Example: A 5'5" woman would have an ideal body-weight range of 113 to 137 pounds. A 5'10" man would have an ideal body-weight range of 149 to 183 pounds.

Crock-Pot Chicken: Easy, Fast, and Flexible

I don't know about you, but I can't wave a magic wand for a delicious home-cooked meal the instant I arrive home with hungry kids in tow.

Here's a quick tip that has helped me pull off a healthy dinner many times:

Put one to two pounds of boneless, skinless chicken breasts in a Crock-Pot and fill the pot about one-third full of water. Let the chicken cook on low for four to eight hours. Make sure the chicken is fully cooked (with no pink meat, clear juices, and a temperature of at least 165 degrees Fahrenheit).

The chicken will be moist and tender, and you can shred it easily so that it's ready to go into any entrée. Try one of these ideas:

- Sprinkle with Mrs. Dash or lemon pepper and serve with a vegetable and some fruit.
- Add taco seasoning and make tacos.
- Add enchilada seasoning and make enchiladas.
- Add to a fresh spinach salad (with slivered almonds, shredded carrots, and tomatoes).
- Add to your favorite casserole dish (brown rice and cream of chicken soup will work).
- Mix with cooked whole-wheat noodles and marinara sauce.

How Much Water during and after Workouts?

A good sweat is part of an effective workout. All that sweat means you are losing water—something you need to remove metabolic by-products, to regulate your body temperature, and to help you keep your energy level up.

Make sure you drink enough water during and after your workouts—today and every day. Here are the simple rules:

1. Drink one cup of water about two hours before you work out.
2. Drink one-half cup about every fifteen minutes during your workout.
3. Drink two to three cups *per pound lost* after your workouts—or drink about one cup of water for every 250 calories you burn.
4. If all this seems too complicated, make it easy: make sure you drink some water before, during, and after your workout today.

Remember, "one cup" is only 8 ounces, which is relatively small. With today's humongous water bottles, it's possible to overhydrate yourself.

Eat Brown Rice Today

For one of your meals today, eat at least one-half cup of brown rice. Brown rice has more fiber, protein, potassium, magnesium, vitamin B$_6$, and zinc than white rice. It has more flavor and texture and keeps you feeling fuller longer. You'll be better off if you can make this wholesome food a part of your regular diet.

Try one of these delicious ways to eat brown rice:

- Use in a casserole.
- Microwave and serve plain with a little salt and pepper.
- Make rice pudding.
- Use as a side dish with meat-and-sauce recipes like meatballs or saucy chicken.
- Combine with a few spoonfuls of canned black beans and a little cheese and salsa and wrap in a whole-wheat tortilla.

If you are eating in a restaurant, ask your server if they have brown rice available as part of your entrée.

Go for a Walk

Go for a walk sometime today. You walk around every day, but today walk with some serious intention. Your objective is to feel refreshed, energized, and healthy. Walk fast enough that your heart is pumping at a steady pace. On a scale of one to ten, with one being little or no effort and ten being maximum effort, you should be walking at a level six to seven. This should feel challenging to hard. You should be able to speak a few words without gasping for air—to ensure you are working at an appropriate intensity level.

If you can recruit your spouse, children, or a friend or neighbor, that's even better. You'll both benefit from working harder and longer—plus, you'll be entertained and have a good time. Use a nearby road or a high school track, indoor mall, neighborhood park, golf course, playing field, or a few city blocks near your office. You can even walk laps around your own house! No excuses. All you need to find is *the time!*

Drop the Salt Shaker

Eat less salt today. Avoid salting your food at the table—and that goes for the car, the restaurant, and the office—everywhere. An innocent "five little shakes" with the salt shaker can quickly add up to one-eighth of a teaspoon of salt. Do that for two items on your plate and you've got one-fourth of a teaspoon. Do that for three items, and you've got about one-half of a teaspoon—or one-half the salt you should eat in an entire day. And you've done it in one meal.

Cutting salt may help control blood pressure, which reduces the risk of stroke (by about 40 percent), heart disease (by about 25 percent), and even dementia.* Salt is present in most of the foods we eat; and very high amounts are included in restaurant foods, boxed meals, and canned goods. But it is found even in healthy foods like milk, breads, and cereals. Try using dried herbs, garlic, or pepper to season your food. Watch out for catch-all seasonings like seasoned salt, onion salt, or steak seasoning; these all contain sodium. Check the label and look for a seasoning with less than 200 mg of sodium per one-fourth teaspoon.

---

*Source: Bonnie Liebman, *Nutrition Action,* vol. 31, no. 3, April 2004 (Center for Science in the Public Interest).

Beta What?

Eat something with beta-carotene today. Beta-carotene is a provitamin that your body converts into vitamin A. It's powerful because it acts as an antioxidant and promotes healthy eyes, growth, bone development, and immune function. Beta-carotene is found in the highest amount in orange, yellow, and leafy green vegetables and fruits.

Eat one of these beta-carotene-rich foods today:

- Sweet potatoes (½ cup, cooked, mashed)
- Canned pumpkin (½ cup, mashed)
- Baby carrots (8–10 each, raw or cooked)
- Mixed vegetables (1 cup, cooked)
- Spinach (1 cup, raw or cooked)
- Sweet red pepper (1 cup, raw or cooked)
- Mango (1 each)
- Papaya (1 each)
- Apricots (3 each)
- Cantaloupe (1 cup)
- Grapefruit (½ each)
- Canned vegetable soup (1 cup, chunky, ready-to-serve)
- Canned vegetable juice (1 cup, low sodium)
- Green peas (1 cup, cooked)
- Broccoli (1 cup, cooked)

Avoiding the "Diet Coke" Syndrome

Picture this: Liz stops at a gas station because she "needs a drink." Her drink has zero calories, and she knows from past experience that the diet soda alone won't calm her craving for a sweet snack. Since the drink has no calories, she goes for it and gets a candy bar to go with that ice cold diet soda.

This scenario (with the person getting either a sweet or a salty snack) is pretty common. It's ironic—the cycle starts with simply needing a drink, but it ends with us eating snacks we wouldn't have eaten in the first place.

If you drink diet soda, fine. But for today (and as many days as you can hereafter), forget about the sweet or salty snacks that you usually also eat. Drink the diet soda by itself or with a healthy snack like sliced apples, a handful of nuts, or a handful of baby carrots. And if that's too easy for you, drop the diet soda altogether and enjoy a glass of water and a healthy snack instead.

Have Your Whole-Grain
Cereal and Eat It, Too

Whatever your issue with whole-grain cereal—if you despise it; don't mind it; like only one kind; or love it, but a member of your family doesn't—try this little trick:

Mix 50 to 75 percent whole-grain cereal with 25 to 50 percent sweetened cereal. This works in a bowl with milk or dry in a snack baggie for on-the-move snacks. The combination of the two cereals makes for interesting new flavors and offers up more nutrition and variety than if you had sworn off the whole-grain cereal altogether. Ideally, you or your family members who take advantage of this "limited time offer" will learn to appreciate and enjoy the taste of 100-percent whole-grain cereal.

Fiber One, Shredded Wheat, Bran Flakes, All-Bran, Kashi Heart to Heart, or Quaker Oatmeal Squares are all high-fiber, whole-grain cereals that mix well with the sweetened cereal of your choice.

Kids and New Foods:
Try, Try, Try Again!

If introducing a new food to your family at the dinner table makes you weak in the knees, read this:

I have a rule to control the "trying new foods" drama. The rule is simple: Be patient. Studies show that it can take up to ten introductions before a child will try a new food. If your child is truly sick at the sight of the new food, don't push it. But if they simply don't want to, "just because," then try, try again. It's a worthy effort if you can instill a lifetime of eating healthy fruits, vegetables, and whole grains (like brown rice, whole-wheat pasta, and high-fiber cereals).

Today, introduce a new healthy food or food that was previously snubbed by your family. Be calm and be patient. Act like it's no big deal if they really don't want to eat the food. Do make them have one taste, and offer positive reinforcement for doing so (read them an extra story, let them go on a quick bike ride, play a quick round of their favorite game after dinner).

Chocolate Cream Dessert— Done Right!

All foods can fit into your life—even chocolate! If you've got a birthday or special event today, try this delicious dessert! It's certainly not an *every-day* food, but it is much improved compared to other desserts out there.

Chocolate Cream Dessert

1 package German chocolate cake mix
1 egg
1 cup applesauce
8 ounces softened, fat-free cream cheese
1 cup powdered sugar
1 cup fat-free whipped topping
1 3.5-ounce package chocolate pudding
1½ cups cold skim milk
3 cups fat-free whipped topping

Mix the cake mix, egg, and applesauce in a medium bowl. Pour into a 9" x 13" pan greased with cooking spray and bake at 350 degrees for 20 minutes.

Mix the cream cheese, powdered sugar, and 1 cup whipped topping together. Spread over the cooled cake. Then mix the pudding and milk; pour over the cream cheese layer.

Spread the remaining 3 cups whipped topping over the top.

The original version, made with real butter and full-fat products, has a whopping 500 calories and 23 grams of fat (15 saturated) per serving. Ouch! But the revised version above is slimmed down to 300 calories and 5 grams of fat (only 2 grams saturated) per serving, which is *much* better. So enjoy!

Butter vs. Margarine: Which Is Best?

Butter is mainly saturated fat. Saturated fat raises our LDL (bad) cholesterol, our risk for obesity, heart disease, and some cancers. Hard stick margarine is a combination of saturated and trans fat (although it's higher in trans fat). Trans fat raises our LDL ("bad") cholesterol and lowers our HDL ("good") cholesterol, which is a double whammy for our health—putting us at an even greater risk for heart disease. Together, trans and saturated fats have officially been blacklisted. They are both bad.

On the other hand, canola-based soft-tub spread (still called margarine in some varieties) consists of healthier monounsaturated fats—which are good for our heart in moderation—with absolutely *no* trans fats.

Thanks to the mandatory nutrition labeling of trans fats in foods, you will now be able to comparison shop for the healthiest fats by simply looking at the label.

The bottom line? You can still keep a stick of butter around for occasional desserts or recipes when you want to go all out—but 80 percent of the time, use the healthier option: *canola-based soft spread or a liquid canola spray.*

Store-Brand Foods: Not Always the Best Buy

Don't worry—this isn't an attempt to make you waste your money and ban all store-brand items. Rather, it's a simple caution to *compare the labels* of store-brand versus name-brand versions on certain foods. Check labels on:

- Yogurt
- Margarine
- Sour cream
- Shortening
- Cereal
- Quick bread mixes (like pancake)

- Breads
- Juice
- Cookies
- Granola bars
- Crackers

The generic or store brand may be cheaper, but it may also have *more* calories, fat, saturated fat, trans fat, sugar, or sodium. This is actually quite common in the food industry. So take five to ten seconds and look at the labels and compare. If it turns out that the brand-name variety is a better nutritional choice, but you don't have the money to spend on it, then think twice about how much you really need the food anyway. If you really need it, just use the cheaper store-brand food in moderation.

TIP #121

A Light Dinner for a Heavy Day

Did you eat an enormous lunch? Maybe it's close to dinner, and you've already snacked on fresh-baked cookies and a glass of milk, or you had a large breakfast *and* lunch so you're thinking your day is already shot. It's not. If you've done any of the above things, realign your day by making a healthy dinner choice. Here's how:

Eat a colorful salad with dark greens and chunks of fresh vegetables for dinner tonight. Use a low-fat dressing, and toss in a few nuts. Add a glass of skim milk or soy milk. If you're still hungry, add a slice of 100-percent whole-grain bread or a few crackers. Don't worry, your body won't starve by eating one light meal; in fact, your body will probably appreciate the light meal so it can clean up the mess you made earlier!

I love all kinds of foods and occasionally eat more than I should. This salad-for-dinner rule of thumb is simple and saves me, time and time again. I know it can work for you as well. Give it a try.

Steam Your Veggies

Some nutrients are absorbed better when the food is raw (like vitamin C in broccoli). Conversely, some nutrients are better absorbed when the food is cooked (like lycopene in tomato products or calcium in leafy greens). That's why you should eat vegetables prepared in different ways for the greatest health benefits, sometimes raw and sometimes cooked.

Steam cooking is the best method to use when you want cooked vegetables. It leaves vegetables lightly crispy and not mushy, brighter in color, and with more of the nutrients intact.

Steam a batch of veggies tonight. It can take as little as five minutes, depending on your preferences. You can use a steaming pot, a wok, or a small kitchen appliance steamer. If steaming is new to you, simply boil some water and place the vegetables in a stainless steel strainer above the boiling water. Cooking with a lid will shorten the cooking time, but will also make the veggies soft and mushy quicker. Cook until the vegetables are tender when pierced with a fork.

TIP #123

The Scoop on Jell-O Salad: Cool Whip and Marshmallows Do Have Calories!

Think of any gelatin or fruit salad. What do almost all of them contain?

Whipped topping, marshmallows, canned fruit—and even crumbled cookies, thanks to a new trend! And where does the fruit or flavored Jell-O (gelatin) that started this dish end up? Smothered.

Don't worry: these sweet, fluffy salads can still fit into your diet in moderation. But today, go for the *plain* version, with chunks of fresh or canned fruit as the topping. Or make a colorful bowl of fresh fruit salad, and skip the whipped topping, skip the marshmallows, and definitely skip the cookies! Doing so cuts the sugar and calories in half and the fat grams to zero.

If you still want to make the whipped topping and marshmallow version of your favorite Jell-O or fruit salad, serve it as a *dessert*—after all, with twenty to thirty grams of sugar (five to seven teaspoons) per serving, that's what it is.

Don't Use "Big" Dishes

If you use a big plate, a big bowl, or a big glass, one thing is bound to happen: you'll serve up a heftier portion than if you had used a smaller-sized plate, dish, or glass. To top it off, having more food sitting in front of us means *we eat more*. It's not a shocking revelation, I know. But it does happen right under our noses every day. Think about the platters (not plates) used by restaurants these days. It's deceiving—we don't feel like we are eating or drinking more than we should because the amount of food looks "normal" in proportion to the large dish.

Today, try to eat foods from smaller plates and bowls and drink beverages from smaller cups. Look in your cupboards. About how much fluid will your "normal" drinking glass hold? My regular glasses hold twelve to sixteen ounces—making it easy for my family to drink a double portion unknowingly. Meanwhile, my teensy *juice glasses* are the perfect size for the eight-ounce recommended serving size for milk, juice, soda pop, and most beverages.

Healthy Chicken Nuggets for Kids

No more fried chicken nuggets! Try these healthy, delicious chicken strips—kids will love them and so will you. They have half the fat, no harmful trans fats, and only one-third of the sodium found in the fast-food versions.

Healthy Chicken Nuggets
1 tablespoon canola oil
⅛ teaspoon salt
¼ teaspoon ground black pepper
1½ cups rolled oats
2 large egg whites
1 pound boneless, skinless chicken breasts

Preheat oven to 450 degrees.

Mix the oil, salt, and pepper in a bowl. Coarsely grind the oats in a blender or food chopper. Whisk the oats and the oil mixture together; then pour into a pie pan. In a separate bowl, whisk the egg whites for one minute.

Cut the chicken breasts into strips. Roll the chicken in the egg whites and then coat well with the oats. Grease a baking sheet with cooking spray. Place the chicken strips on a baking sheet, and then coat them with cooking spray.

Bake 15 to 18 minutes, until the chicken is tender and golden brown. Let cool on the baking sheet for 3 to 5 minutes.

Nutrients per 2 strips: 180 calories, 5 grams fat, 1 gram saturated fat, 160 mg sodium, 2 grams fiber, 21 grams protein.

Grilled-Cheese Sandwiches: Try the Healthier Version

"A little sandwich with no meat and no mayo has got to be lower in fat than a cheeseburger!" Nope.

A restaurant-prepared grilled-cheese sandwich can harbor about 600 calories and 30 grams of fat—similar to the amount found in a *double* cheeseburger. The problem? Two slices of bread coated in butter, and a thick layer of gooey cheese.

I'm a bad cook, so grilled cheese makes a regular appearance on the Douglass menu. Here's how I make grilled cheese healthier in my own home. It works well for us—give it a try for you and your family today.

1. Skip the butter. If you prefer your sandwich a little crispier, briefly spray the pan with cooking spray.
2. Use wheat bread.
3. Don't overload with cheese: use only two slices of processed cheese or a ¼-inch thick slice of block cheese.

With about 400 calories and 10 grams of fat per sandwich, this healthier version will be more kind to your arteries.

Wash Those Hands!

Wash your hands today. Be conscientious. Don't put anything in your mouth unless you've washed your hands first. This might be a little extreme for everyday living, but hopefully you'll find some middle ground where you *usually* wash your hands before eating, touching your mouth, nose, or eyes, or touching dishes or utensils. Hand washing lessens the risk of contracting contagious illnesses or coming in contact with potentially life-threatening bacteria. It also decreases the risk of you spreading an illness to those around you.

Wash your hands *immediately* after you:

- Touch raw meat, poultry, or fish.
- Touch raw egg shells, whites, or yolks.
- Touch cookie dough, cake batters, or other mixtures that contain raw, unpasteurized eggs.
- Touch garbage.
- Change diapers.
- Use the bathroom.
- Cough, sneeze, or blow your nose.

The Proper Order of Beverage Drinking

Drink the healthiest beverages first today. For example, water before milk, milk before juice, and juice before soda. You don't have to drink all the healthy beverages in the morning and all the unhealthy beverages in the evening. Rather, if you sit down for lunch and want a glass of lemonade, drink a nice, cold glass of water before drinking the lemonade.

Here's the ideal order of beverage drinking, from the healthiest to the not-so-healthy option.

1. Water
2. Low-fat milk
3. 100-percent juice
4. Sweetened fruit drinks or lemonades
5. Soda pop (diet or regular)

By drinking the most nutrient-dense beverage first (or purest beverage, in the case of water), you'll quench your thirst and fill up your stomach so that you are less inclined to load up on the empty-calorie, non-nutritive beverages later. As a rule of thumb, count 100 calories per eight-ounce cup of beverage (except water and diet soda).

TIP #129

Don't Fall for "0 Grams Trans Fat"

I went to the grocery store today and counted at least five different brands of cookies that stated "0 grams trans fat!" right on the front of the package. That's right—cookies.

Just because a food has no trans fat, does that make it healthy? The answer is a resounding *no!* Saturated fat and trans fat are equally harmful to our health. So a food can claim "0 grams trans fat" on a label while still hosting enough saturated fat and calories to give your ticker a run for its money.

Today, pledge to yourself that you will not fall for the "0 grams trans fat" trick. It doesn't automatically mean a food is good for you. Review the label to make sure the food isn't high in fat (no more than 3 grams per 100 calories) or saturated fat (no more than 1 gram per 100 calories). Your heart will appreciate the effort.

TIP #130

Don't Label Others as Fat, Skinny, Healthy, or Unhealthy

It can be intentional or unintentional or so second nature that it happens unknowingly. With a single judgmental word, our society often looks at others and automatically puts them into a category. Words like "fat," "overweight," "obese," "skinny," "healthy," "fit," "lazy," or "unhealthy" are often used to classify others. It's unfortunate.

Today, don't judge, label, or classify a single soul. Whoever you come into contact with, look into their eyes first, notice their smile, or engage them in a conversation so your impressions of that person can be based on their *character* and not their *looks*. They could be trying just as hard—or harder—than you to have a strong and healthy body. We all deserve better.

This is an uphill battle for sure, and we have a long way to go. Our society is *finally* starting to realize that health isn't about how you look, but it's about how you live. You don't have to be a size six to be happy, healthy, and wise. Rather, you need to be active, eat healthy most of the time, and feel good about yourself and those whom you interact with.

Fitness Test: Walk a Mile

Here's an uncomplicated way to help you test your fitness level and monitor your progress. Take this quick fitness test today.

1. Find a watch, stopwatch, or some sort of timer.
2. Warm up by marching in place or walking at a moderate pace for three to five minutes.
3. Time yourself as you walk a full mile as fast as you can. How long did it take you? Write down the date and the time it took you to walk that distance. Be exact, down to the second.
4. Repeat the test every four to six weeks to monitor progress. (Your goal is to shorten your time.)

Nothing is more depressing than working out and not seeing a visual benefit. Sometimes those visual benefits take longer than we expect; sometimes they never meet our expectations. But the *real* benefit of exercise always happens on the inside. As you shorten your time, that means your body is pumping more blood with each heartbeat, moving more oxygen through your lungs with every breath, and generating more power from more efficient muscles.

Enjoy Some Popcorn with That Movie!

If you don't like movie-theater popcorn, this tip is not for you. Skip this one. I don't want to taint you by *recommending* that you actually partake of this addicting food! But if you do crave (and regularly partake of) movie-theater popcorn, here's how you can do so on a smaller scale—in other words, healthfully.

Eat the popcorn two to three kernels at a time during the movie. It will last longer.

Got that? (There had better be no excuses that "the popcorn rule" was too hard to remember!)

Instead of shoveling in handful after handful and barely tasting it, take time to enjoy it and eat it *slowly*. By eating two to three kernels at a time, you might end up eating about three to four cups of popcorn during a movie—maybe even less. That's a lot better than the ten to twenty cups you can consume when grabbing huge handfuls of popcorn.

Sweets Served Last

My mom always told me "no sugar before dinner." But as soon as I was on my own, I threw that rule out the window. Until now, that is. Trying to get my kids to eat healthier foods has made me rethink things. And guess what? Big shocker—my mom was right.

I've always loved all foods—fruits, vegetables, whole grains, and all. So for me it wasn't a big deal to eat a cookie before dinner. The cookie never ruined my appetite for healthy foods because I loved those just as much; in fact, I gobbled them up as fast as the cookie. But I was naive. Not everybody loves the taste of fruits, vegetables, and whole grains—especially kids growing up with a highly processed food supply like ours.

Today, make sure you save all sweet-tasting foods for last—not the last of the day, but the last of the meal or snack. Even save sweet fruits for last. Sweet flavors really can make normally accepted vegetables or whole grains taste odd and unappetizing.

What's Your BMI?

This tip works in combination with tip #108. It's important to look at all factors that affect your health. Your eating habits, your exercise habits, your genes, your body weight, your body fat percentage, and your Body Mass Index (BMI) are all key components in determining your health status and risk for disease. BMI is a simple screening for weight categories that may lead to health problems. It's *one part* of the big picture.

Today, calculate your BMI. You can do this in two ways:

1. *The old-fashioned way.* Plug your height and weight into the following calculation:

   Take your weight (in pounds), divide by your height (in inches) squared; then multiply by 703 [weight (pounds) ÷ height (inches)^2 x 703]. The answer is your BMI.

   Example: If you weigh 200 pounds and are 65 inches tall, then 200 x 4225 = .0473 x 703 = 33.3.

2. *The computer way.* Visit http://www.cdc.gov and type in this search: "BMI calculator." It's downright easy to use and will take thirty seconds!

The standard categories associated with BMI are as follows:

BMI	Weight Status
Less than 18.5	Underweight
18.5–24.9	Normal
25.0–29.9	Overweight
More than 30.0	Obese

Hoodia Hype

The latest "lose-weight-fast miracle potion" is out in full force. It's called hoodia, and it's all over the Internet and in retail stores nationwide.

Hoodia is a plant from South Africa that can act as an appetite suppressant. Only one *small* study has ever been done on humans, and it has yet to be published. We don't have a clue what the side effects are and how often or how much hoodia can be consumed safely.

If you're thinking about diet pills, or if you currently take them, don't waste your valuable money on hoodia-based ones (read the ingredients). The hoodia plant grows only in the South African desert and takes *years* to reach full maturity, which makes you wonder—how are all these manufacturers selling products with hoodia when it is outright scarce? Well, apparently they're not. It seems much of the hoodia sold in the United States isn't even hoodia at all. On December 13, 2005, *The Wall Street Journal** reported that ten samples of hoodia products were tested and none of them contained a substantial amount of the miraculous hoodia.

This scenario is all too common when it comes to weight-loss pills, supplements, and herbal quick-fix products. So be a conscientious consumer when it comes to these kinds of products.

---

*Source: Dr. James J. Kenney, PhD, RD, FACN, in
http://www.pritikin.com/askexperts/007.shtml.

TIP #136

The Law of the Fats

Some fats are good; some are bad. The typical American eats more than enough fat, so while we need to eat less fat in general, we also need to *replace* the bad fats with the good. So don't *add* fat to your diet today. The average American needs about sixty to ninety grams of fat per day. No more than twenty grams should be from those harmful saturated or trans fats. Today, choose the healthy fats over the unhealthy fats; it will help you make room for the good fats and squeeze out those insidious bad fats.

Bad Fats (Don't eat these today)	Good Fats or Replacements (Do eat these today)
Butter	Peanut butter, soft canola spread, or canola oil cooking spray
Cheese	Nuts (all kinds; 1–2 ounces only)
Vegetable shortening or margarine	Canola, olive, peanut, or safflower oils
Sour cream	Guacamole
Red meat	Fatty fish like salmon or trout
Fried foods	Baked foods (not cake, cookies, white bread)
Crackers or chips	Pretzels or whole-wheat toast
Cookies or sweets	Peppermint candies or fruit (dried or fresh)
Whole or 2% milk	1% or nonfat milk

TIP #137

Don't Be a Meal Skipper

If you regularly skip breakfast and/or lunch and then enjoy a nice, big dinner, read up. This one's for you.

Skipping a meal *from time to time* can be an effective way to balance your calorie intake—but this shouldn't happen more than once per week. You don't "eat less" when skipping meals is your daily routine.

The Life of a Meal Skipper

Lori skips breakfast and has a granola bar for lunch. She gets home at about 5:30 P.M., completely famished! She pours a glass of lemonade and eats three handfuls of wheat crackers. While she prepares dinner, she nibbles on two handfuls of M&Ms and some baby carrots. She then eats a dinner of chicken, rice, steamed veggies, fruit salad, and two rolls with butter—after all, she hasn't eaten all day. Just before bed, she has a dish of ice cream and a tall glass of water.

Guess how many calories she just ate. It's 2600—all of it eaten after 5:30 P.M.

Your goal today: Eat three sensible meals. You'll end up eating about the same (or fewer) calories *in healthily spaced increments* instead of all at once.

Quick and Easy Whole-Wheat Waffles

Wholesome, nutritious waffles are easier than you think. Whole-wheat waffles are a good source of fiber, and even though they contain fat, they offer up healthier monounsaturated fats. Try these today:

Whole-Wheat Waffles

1 egg
1¾ cups skim milk
¼ cup canola oil
2 cups 100-percent whole-wheat flour
1 tablespoon baking powder
¼ teaspoon salt

Whisk the egg, milk, and oil together in a medium bowl. Then add the flour, baking powder, and salt, and mix thoroughly. (These waffles turn out just fine even when the ingredients are thrown together all at once, just in case you are into fast, easy, and use-fewer-dishes cooking—like me.)

Pour the batter onto a hot waffle iron lightly greased with cooking spray. Bake until done. Makes 9 waffles.

Nutrients per waffle: 120 calories, 5 grams fat, 1 gram saturated fat, 2 grams fiber, 2 grams protein.

Give Food a Second Chance

If you avoid a certain food "because I don't like that!" try giving it a second chance today. (Of course, don't ever eat anything to which you are allergic.) This rule applies to healthy foods such as vegetables, fruits, whole grains, low-fat dairy or soy products, and beans, nuts, or seeds. Wanting a healthy body and believing that a certain food can give you that benefit can make the taste and texture of food quickly become tolerable—and soon even likable. Your mind is that powerful.

Most of us are a little spoiled when it comes to food. We expect our food to be superb and delicious and to hit the spot *every meal of every day.* Nothing wrong there—food should be enjoyed. But look around: what kinds of choices are we making day after day? Are people buying bags of fruits and vegetables from the drive-thru? Calling restaurants to deliver brown rice and baked chicken? Not in this world. Think about it—our taste buds need some reacclimation and variety, so give one of those neglected healthy foods a second chance today.

Don't Buy Foods That Taunt You

Back when we thought fat-free everything was our ticket to permanent good health, I had a tiny addiction to red licorice. I kept buying it, and then getting mad at myself for eating too much of it. But one day as I walked down the grocery store aisle, I did something that made the temptation disappear: I turned my head and *walked away.* Seems simple enough, right? If it tempts you, don't buy it. Don't even look at it. And certainly don't make it a part of your weekly grocery list. Once in a while, fine. But if you buy tempting foods *you will eat them!* (Now try to make sense of that . . .)

Whatever your temptation today—a bakery, a grocery store aisle full of cookies, or a vending machine with chocolate—just don't buy it. If you can make it through that, the rest is easy. You can't eat what isn't sitting in front of you. Distract your mind with another activity so you can move on to other, more important things.

New Exercise Move: The Plank

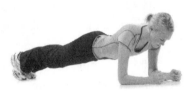

A plank is a balancing position you hold for ten to thirty seconds at a time. This exercise mainly strengthens your abdominals but works your entire body as well, thanks to the total body stabilization that is needed (and developed) with this exercise.

Find a soft towel and get down on the floor on your hands and knees. Fold the towel over and place it under your hands. Now drop your elbows, and let them rest on the towel. Extend your legs straight back behind you and balance on your toes. Make sure your elbows are directly below your shoulders and your legs are straight. Your abs should be tightly contracted (pull your belly button up toward your spine), your glutes should be contracted, and your shoulders should be pulled back (don't let your shoulders round toward the floor). Hold this position for ten to thirty seconds—breathing in and out in a controlled manner as you hold. Then drop to the floor and rest for thirty seconds. Repeat this exercise two to three more times.

Music: Powerful Workout Fuel

Try some music to help you get through your workout today. Not only does music provide a refreshing new motivation for working out, but it also makes it more fun, more exciting, and more efficient! Honestly, I would be bored to tears and make it no more than five minutes without some heart-pumping tunes to keep me going. Music gives me focus, determination, stamina, willpower, and so much more. It really is my lifesaver—my *source of energy* for staying fit and healthy in this noisy, busy world.

Music with a steady 125 to 145 beats per minute works well for most forms of exercise. Find music you enjoy, but make sure it's upbeat and steady so you can move to the beat.

Not all music makes perfect "workout music." Visit www.power music.com—the masters of workout music. They've certainly harnessed the extraordinary power of music and have a substantial offering of inspiring music engineered specifically for working out.

Eating at an Amusement Park? Then Pat the Fat

Are you visiting an amusement park, water park, sporting event, or even the county fair? If so, chances are good you'll end up being surrounded by tempting food, and with a hungry stomach to boot. I'm not advocating the consumption of greasy foods by any means, but this advice can at least help lessen the offense to your poor arteries when placed in this environment.

Pizza, chicken strips, nuggets, fries, corn dogs, cheesy breadsticks, hot dogs, even hamburger patties—all these foods are "patable." You can pat the food with a clean paper towel or napkin to absorb unwanted grease and fat. You can even go past "patting"; wrap a napkin around it and squeeze it! Every little bit *and drop* of fat you *don't* eat is beneficial for your health.

If you order a big cookie, pastry, or cinnamon roll, let it sit on a napkin for about five minutes to absorb some grease and fat. Then *share* the probably oversized treat with a friend and enjoy the rest of your day without "rock-gut" (my term for queasy stomachs thanks to sugar, grease, large portions, and fast, adrenaline-pumping rides).

Stop and *Taste* the Food

I'm all for enjoying your favorite foods in moderation. I am not, however, a fan of eating your favorite foods so fast (or while you are so busy) that you completely miss out on the enjoyment of the food. What is the point of making your body deal with a bunch of excess calories when you didn't even taste it—or worse, didn't even *notice* that you ate it?

Stop, sit down, and actually *taste* the food you eat today. If you slip up and start to mindlessly eat food, then make yourself sit down—or stop what you are doing—and take two minutes to eat the food in peace. If you give your brain a chance to send the "I'm satisfied" signals, it will. Those signals are essential to having a healthy relationship with food. Enjoy a small amount of your favorite food *with intention,* and then move on with your day. Get busy crossing other important things off your to-do list.

Hip Flexors: Stretch Them Out!

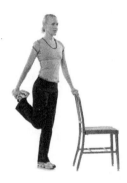

Sit down in a chair and press your fingers into the crease between your upper leg and your hip bones—those are your hip flexors. And because we tend to sit through most of the day, they are likely very tight—so tight, in fact, that they can cause your entire pelvis to tilt forward, which can then force your lower back to be in an arched position, which can then cause back pain, muscular imbalances, and potential back injuries.

Stretch your hip flexors today. Stand next to a chair in a perpendicular position (with the left side of your body facing the chair). Place your left hand on the chair for balance. Lift your right foot off the floor and bring the heel toward your glutes. Grab the foot with your right hand; keep your right knee pointing toward the floor and press your foot *away from your body* by pushing the foot against your hand. Now deepen the stretch by pressing your right hip slightly forward. Hold the stretch for twenty to thirty seconds. Then perform the stretch with the left leg.

Sodium Swap: Simple Tricks You Can't Miss

Check this out:

Prepared Food	Sodium (mg)
Cheesy chicken with pasta (meal in a box)	930
Whole-wheat pasta	0
Boxed rice with seasoning	1070
Boxed rice with ½ packet seasoning	535
Brown rice with a dash of salt and pepper	150
Cheeseburger macaroni ("Just Add Hamburger"meal)	910
Hamburger with steamed veggies and fruit	150
Canned vegetables	350
Fresh vegetables	0
Regular canned soup	800–1000
"Healthy" labeled soup	less than 480
"Low Sodium" soup	less than 140

Remember, we should eat only 1500 to 2300 mg of sodium per day. The lower sodium alternatives should be clear to see. Make a healthy sodium swap today. In general, avoid canned and boxed foods. If you must use a boxed food, use only half of the flavoring or sauce packet (that's where most of the sodium is hiding). Fresh and plain is always a good thing when it comes to sodium!

Lost Your Motivation?
It's Right Here

We all go through this. Feeling overwhelmed, feeling like you're not up to par, feeling tired, or just plain ready to give up. It's a natural part of the ebb and flow of life. But if you want to change your health for a lifetime, it's something you have to work on for a lifetime. All you need to do is be willing to try, try again. Try one of these tips to help you get back on the right path:

- Talk to a positive friend. The conversation doesn't even have to be about you. Hearing a positive spin on life is always inspiring.
- Listen to your favorite music.
- Invite a friend or family member to work out with you. Set a time and date—and don't cancel it!
- Invite somebody to enjoy a healthy meal with you. The invitation will force you to follow through with making and eating the healthy meal.
- Ponder your true intentions. Tell yourself you "have" to do it in order to feel your best. You have no choice other than to fight for your health in this unhealthy world.

Movie Night . . . with Healthy Snacks!

Watch a movie with your family tonight. There is one rule, however: you have to serve healthy snacks. Seriously, your body will appreciate it! When you barely move a muscle for two hours and top it off by eating a bunch of high-calorie food, your poor body has to find a place to use or store all those extra calories.

Here's to the healthiest movie-watching experience of your life. Try one or two of these ideas:

- *A bowl of mixed fresh fruit:* grapes, cantaloupe, berries, and so forth
- *Plain popcorn:* with a dash of salt and *a little* spray butter
- *Veggie tray:* dip with ranch dressing, but not sour-cream-based ranch dip
- *One portion of one treat per person:* one-quarter cup M&Ms, two small cookies, and so forth (allow one portion; then put the rest away—out of sight)
- *Hard candies:* try four to six per person (they take longer to eat and can satisfy a sweet tooth with a small amount of calories)
- *Sugar-free frozen yogurt:* skip the ten to twelve teaspoons of sugar in regular frozen yogurt
- *Ice water*

Fruit and Yogurt

Try dipping your favorite fruit in some plain or vanilla low-fat yogurt. Melons, berries, mangos, kiwi, apple, or banana slices and almost any fruit are all delicious when dipped in creamy, calcium-rich yogurt.

Watch out for ready-made "fruit dip" products and fruited yogurts that tend to be high in calories, thanks to nine to ten teaspoons of sugar in just a half-cup serving. Here are the best yogurt dips, ranked in order from least calories and sugar to the most. Serving size is one-half cup, unless otherwise noted.

Yogurt	Calories	Sugar (g)
Plain nonfat yogurt	50	6.5
Vanilla light yogurt	60	7.5
Plain lowfat yogurt	80	9
Vanilla lowfat yogurt	110	19
Strawberry fruit dip	120*	14
Fruited lowfat yogurt	120	21
Chocolate fruit dip	220*	18

Fruit parfaits make great refreshments for parties, family get-togethers, and church activities. Mix fresh fruit, plain yogurt, and a few scoops of some high-fiber granola for a delicious treat or snack.

---

*Per one-fourth cup

Open Sesame: Kiwi Peeling Made Easy

A kiwi is one of the healthiest fruits you can eat. Yet many people don't. The common excuse I hear is that "they are too hard to peel." Time to cross that barrier off the list. Here's an easy way to peel a kiwi:

Take a knife and barely cut the top stem area off. Then grab one of your kitchen spoons and wedge it between the skin and flesh of the kiwi. Slowly rotate the kiwi and lift the skin away from the flesh. Press the spoon up toward the flesh as you rotate the kiwi. You should be able to peel the entire kiwi in one easy rotation. When you're done, just cut the kiwi in half and slice it like an orange.

Eat some kiwi today. They are cheap, convenient, and healthy. Two fresh kiwi fruit supply more than *an entire day's* worth of vitamin C. You'll also get as much fiber as is found in two slices of 100-percent whole-wheat bread, as well as a good dose of folate, magnesium, potassium, vitamin K, and copper.

TIP #151

What's Coming Up This Week?

Take a minute to think about what you have on your schedule for this upcoming week. Do you have a birthday party? A day with not-a-spare-minute for cooking a decent meal? Write down the problematic days for you. How can you balance the day? Here are a few examples of how you can plan ahead to avoid total food and activity meltdowns.

1. Birthday party, Wednesday, 5:00 P.M. . . .
   Have a vigorous workout at 6:30 A.M. and eat a light lunch: a salad with some soup or wheat bread.
2. Busy day, Thursday, all day (work till 4:00 P.M., piano lessons at 4:30, then softball game at 6:00) . . .
   Run on the treadmill for twenty minutes first thing in the morning. Leave the house with snacks: apples, wheat crackers, string cheese, and bottled water. Put chicken in the crockpot so dinner is ten-minutes-from-ready when we arrive home.
3. Cookout with friends, Saturday at 7:00 P.M. . . .
   Take the kids for a bike ride at 8:00 A.M.; don't eat any sweets all day—my sweets allotment for the day is going to be saved for two delicious s'mores!

"So What Exactly Should I Eat?"

If I had a dime for every time somebody asked, "So can you just give me a meal plan? I don't want to figure it out—just tell me what to eat," I'd be a rich woman. I agree that seeing an ideal "healthy" menu for a day is helpful. So here's a good example of a dietitian's "dream day"—which has fruits, vegetables, at least 25 grams of fiber, not too much fat or sugar, and a modest 1800 calories. Humor me, and try to eat something close to this today.

Breakfast
- 1 cup Bran Flakes
- 1 cup skim milk
- ½ cup raspberries

Morning Snack
- 10–15 baby carrots
- 1 ounce string cheese
- 1 glass water

Lunch
- 2 cups leafy greens
- ½ cup canned kidney or black beans
- ½ tomato
- 2 tablespoons sliced almonds
- ¼ cup low-fat salad dressing
- 1 whole-wheat roll
- 2 teaspoons jam
- 1 glass water or diet beverage

Afternoon Snack
- 1 apple
- 4 hard candies or bite-sized chocolates
- 1 glass water

Dinner
- 3 ounces grilled or baked chicken
- ½ cup brown rice
- 1 cup steamed broccoli
- 1 cup skim milk

Evening Snack
- 1 orange
- 1 chewy granola bar

Use Your Dinner Table

Make it a priority to eat dinner at the table *and as a family* tonight. Eating at the dinner table means you're more likely to:

- Serve and eat a balanced meal.
- Enjoy much-needed family time.
- Listen to *and hear* what your kids have to say.
- Eat and chew your food more slowly (you'll feel more full faster, even when you've actually eaten less food than normal).

And you'll be less likely to:

- Snack before dinner (knowing that a structured meal is soon to be served).
- Swallow large amounts of unchewed food, which can be hard to digest.
- Mindlessly eat foods that you don't even like, want, or need.

Don't forget to delegate; assign other members of the family to help set the table, prepare certain food items, and wash the dishes. These days, it's too daunting to serve family meals at a dinner table when you are the one who has to do all the work! If it's a group effort, the meal time is beneficial to all.

How to Burn More Calories While You Walk

For some, walking is too easy: "not intense enough," they say. For some, running is too hard: "It hurts my knees." For those people and everyone in between, walking *on an incline* is the answer.

Walking on an incline (going uphill) can burn up to three times the calories of the average casual walk on a level surface. You'll work and sweat harder without all the painful impact to your knees and joints. Walking on an incline can also define and strengthen problem areas: those stubborn hips, glutes, and thighs. Here are a few great ways to walk on an incline:

- Find an uphill mountain or nature trail.
- Walk on an uphill sidewalk or road.
- Use a treadmill with an incline.*

Go for a thirty-minute uphill walk today. If you don't have thirty minutes to spare, try it for ten minutes—anything counts! I just want you to feel the "incline difference." Bend your arms to a 90-degree angle and pump them forward and back as you walk. As always, listen to your body and work at a challenging, but comfortable pace.

---

*Visit www.proform.com or www.nordictrack.com for more information on treadmills with incline.

Banana Splits for Dessert!

We all like sweets once in a while (it makes me feel better to acknowledge that I'm not the only one who needs a little chocolate now and then!), so today, satisfy your sweet tooth with a healthy banana split. It's easy—all you need are:

Banana Splits

1 banana

2–3 tablespoons low-fat yogurt, regular or frozen (or low-fat whipped topping)

2–3 tablespoons fresh or frozen berries

1 tablespoon nuts (your favorite kind)

A drizzle of chocolate or caramel syrup

Slice a banana lengthwise (you can keep it in the peel or place it in a dish). Top the banana with the yogurt (low-fat plain, or light vanilla is best) or whipped topping (fat-free, low-fat is best). Then top the banana with the berry of your choice (strawberries, raspberries, or blueberries are delightful) and a few nuts. Drizzle a small amount of chocolate or caramel syrup—but think of the syrup as a "garnish," not a topping! Make a skinny zigzag and call it good.

Vitamin Savvy: Get Your Iron in Today

Iron is an important nutrient that carries oxygen to every cell in your body so those cells can produce energy. If you're low on iron, you can feel tired and weak, and have intolerance to cold temperatures.

The iron found in meat, poultry, or fish is called heme iron; it is absorbed and used very efficiently by the body. (That's one good reason to eat a small amount of meat in your diet.) The iron found in plant foods like leafy greens and beans isn't absorbed as well as the heme iron found in meats. You can also get iron from enriched or fortified foods, such as cold cereal, breads, bagels, and other flour-based products.

The best thing to do is eat a variety and consume vitamin-C-rich foods (because vitamin C helps your body absorb iron). Make sure you consume at least one of these iron-rich foods today:

- 1 cup cold cereal
- 2 slices whole-grain bread
- 3 ounces lean beef, poultry, or fish
- 2 cups spinach or other dark, leafy greens
- ½ to 1 cup cooked beans

Eating Lunch or Dinner in a Restaurant Today?

Order skinless baked chicken, salad with dressing on the side, and brown rice, whole-wheat pasta, or steamed vegetables. If you don't want chicken, order a broth-based soup—preferably with beans, lentils, or chunks of vegetables.

Compare the restaurant meals below.* (You don't have to ban all restaurant food, but it's always good to be aware of what you are putting into your body—so you can make up for it later with a healthier choice. Restaurant entrees would be half as offensive if the restaurant served half the portion size.)

Menu Item	Calories (Daily goal = 2000–2200)	Fat (g) (Daily goal = less than 65 grams)	Sodium (mg) (Daily goal = less than 2300 mg)
Fettuccine Alfredo (2½ cups)	1500	97	1030
Kung Pao chicken (3 cups) with rice (1⅓ cups) and an egg roll	1275	62	2209
Chicken enchiladas (5 ounces) with refried beans and rice	1260	57	2850
Sirloin steak (12 ounces) with Caesar salad and baked potato with butter	1100	58	1330

Menu Item	Calories (Daily goal = 2000–2200)	Fat (g) (Daily goal = less than 65 grams)	Sodium (mg) (Daily goal = less than 2300 mg)
Fried shrimp (7 ounces) with rice pilaf (1 cup) and one roll or biscuit	920	37	2090
Country-fried steak (9 ounces) with vegetables (1 cup) and mashed potatoes with gravy (¾ cup)	900	52	1990
Ham and pineapple pizza (2 slices)	620	30	1780
Steak and cheese 6″ sub with a snack bag of potato chips	590	28	1470
Baked chicken breast (10 ounces) with salad (2 table-spoons fat-free dressing) and vegetable	550	14	1150

*Source: M. F. Jacobson and J. G. Hurley, *Restaurant Confidential* (New York: Workman Publishing, 2002) and USDA Agricultural Research Service Nutrient Database for Standard Reference, Release 18.

11 Healthy Snacks Sure to Calm a Craving

Try one of these great snacks to calm a craving for a high-calorie, high-sugar, or high-fat food. All of these snacks have some serious satisfying power. They really do taste good and can hold your appetite over until you can eat a nutritious, filling meal.

- Orville Redenbacher's Caramel Popcorn Cake topped with one tablespoon peanut butter
- Skinny Cow ice cream treat
- Sugar-free frozen fruit popsicle
- One packet All-Bran Snack Bites (my favorite—very delicious!)
- One cup low-fat frozen yogurt with fresh berries (small size)
- Baked corn chips with salsa
- Three to four cups plain popcorn with a little spray butter and salt
- A handful of nuts and one ounce string cheese
- A slice of whole-wheat toast with jam
- One cup whole-grain cereal with sliced bananas and low-fat milk
- Three to four hard peppermint candies

Sleep Tight . . . All Night

Get eight hours of sleep tonight. Sleep is often ignored as a vital part of "taking care of our bodies." But it shouldn't be. Our bodies need that restful time to rejuvenate, to repair, and to be free of stimulation. You don't even have to be tired, stressed, or scatterbrained to deserve a good night's rest.

In an ideal world, you'd get a good seven to eight hours of sleep every night. But who lives in an ideal world, right? With three children under the age of six, I often end up staying up late or getting up very early because that's my one and only chance for some peaceful and productive quiet time. But I never burn the midnight oil on consecutive nights. If you cheat yourself out of a good night's rest, follow it up the next night with a good seven to eight hours of sleep. Getting a mere four to six hours of sleep shouldn't be a routine; instead, it should be a once-in-a-while occurrence. It's simply not healthy to steal that restful, rejuvenating time from your already hard-working body.

TIP #160

Keep Your Sanity with Guilt-Free Dinners

I think many of us feel that we have to make something extravagant for dinner each day. And feeling that "there's nothing *good* to cook for dinner" can be the one driving factor that, well, ends up driving us out the door—and to the nearest restaurant. So get rid of the guilt by letting go of the idea of a "perfect dinner." Adjust your standards to make your priorities be (1) nutrition, (2) ease, and (3) taste. Here are three downright easy dinners that nourish your body and will keep your sanity intact. Try one today!

Dinner Option 1

Fresh fruit; steamed veggies (or veggies with salad dressing dip); whole-wheat toast with cheese or peanut butter; low-fat milk.

Dinner Option 2

Boiled eggs over fresh baby spinach (or greens) topped with tomatoes, green peas (microwave frozen peas for one minute to soften), carrots, corn, or any vegetables of choice; low-fat salad dressing; fruit; low-fat milk.

Dinner Option 3

Canned beans wrapped in tortillas (whole-wheat) with a sprinkle of cheese and salsa; apple slices or fresh berries; low-fat milk.

162

Give Up Something Good for Something Better

If choosing not to partake of a certain food for health reasons ever makes you feel that you are being deprived or shortchanged, think: "Give up something good for something better." Seriously. Imprint this on your mind right now; repeat it to yourself ten times. I want this encouraging thought to be fresh on your mind and ready to strengthen you in a moment of weakness.

For example, if you choose to have only one slice of pizza (with a salad) instead of three heavy slices, you'll get something better: you won't feel sick and uncomfortable from eating too much. Or if you sacrifice thirty minutes of extra sleep so you can start your morning with some heart-pumping exercise, you'll get something better: more energy and focus to help you through the day.

There are countless rewards that come from giving up something good for something *profoundly* better: feeling stronger; controlling blood pressure and cholesterol levels (a.k.a., silent killers); reducing the risk of disease; feeling happy, less stressed, and more emotionally stable; and most important, having a healthy body that allows you to do the things you love to do.

Mini-Sized Watermelon: Good or Bad?

The answer is definitely good! Thanks to the new mini-sized watermelon, there's no reason not to enjoy luscious watermelon on a regular basis (in season). You don't have to lug a huge, heavy watermelon out of the store, you don't have to cut and slice loads of watermelon that may end up getting wasted or spoiled, and you don't have to find an entire spare shelf in your fridge to store the cut watermelon.

Contrary to popular belief, watermelon is not "just water," and the mini size packs just as much nutritional value as the large size. Watermelon is one of the best food sources of lycopene (a powerful antioxidant that can help fight or prevent disease) and just two cups of juicy watermelon supply a hefty dose of lycopene and beta-carotene, along with vitamin C, potassium, and fiber. The price for a mini watermelon is reasonable; and when you add in the fact that you won't be wasting as much and that it's more convenient and functional, it's definitely worth the price.

Try a mini watermelon today.

Feel Like You've Tried and Failed?

Do you feel like you have tried and failed over and over again to change your health habits? Do you feel like you are at an utter standstill?

Think "simple" today. You know you have to eat less sugar and eat more fruits and vegetables. You know that you have to move your muscles if you want to keep them. Right? Okay, here's how to get yourself going again—on the right foot:

1. Set a specific, realistic goal. "I want to exercise for at least twenty minutes on Monday, Wednesday, and Friday this week."

2. Write it down—place the note somewhere that will be visible on a daily basis. Your closet door, your fridge, or your computer keyboard work well.

3. Expect that you may lapse in some way—it may be for a day, an entire week, or even several weeks. That's normal.

4. Realize that you can have a *fresh start* at any moment you choose. You will always succeed in some capacity—as long as you get back on the right path and try, try again.

Going Camping? Learn to Balance the Classic Campout Meal

A simple meal during a family campout such as a hot dog with cheese on a bun, a few potato chips, two s'mores, and a can of soda pop, lemonade, or fruit punch can have a whopping 1000 calories, 48 grams of fat, 66 grams of sugar (about 17 teaspoons), and 1400 mg of sodium—all too high for the *third* meal of the day.

Here are five simple things that won't wreck all the fun—but that can make your next campout meal a little bit healthier. Try one or all of these today:

- Drop the sugary beverage. Drink diet versions or water.
- Drop the cheese on the hamburger or hot dog.
- Serve sliced fresh fruit or baked corn chips instead of regular chips.
- Don't serve too many items. The more macaroni, potato, and/or fruit salads you serve, the more people eat. Pick one or none.
- Eat one s'more and call it good. Eat more fruit if you still have a craving for something sweet.

New Exercise Move:
Reverse Lunge

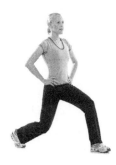 Sculpt and strengthen your legs with this fun lunge:

Stand on a bottom stair (or one stair above the floor) and face the staircase so that you have about five feet of empty space behind you. Feet should be hip width apart with toes pointing forward. Now, step your right foot back and down to the floor and about two to three feet behind you; lower your body until your front knee (left) is bent to a 90-degree angle. Keep your front knee directly above the ankle—don't let it jet forward! Now, lift your body up and bring the right leg back up to starting position. For the other leg: step your left foot back and down to the floor behind you; lower your body until your front knee (right) is bent to a 90-degree angle. Keep that front knee directly above the ankle. Now, lift your body up and bring the left leg back up to starting position.

March in place for one to three minutes, then do two sets of ten to twenty-five reps. Listen to your body and work at your own pace. A slow and controlled pace is always best.

Beginner: You can do this without the stair and just step back on the floor.

Advanced: You can stand on the second stair so that you are lunging back from two stairs instead of one.

Nature Walk

Go for a walk today on a nature-encompassed trail in a shady, green park, in the mountains, or in your favorite scenic area. The beauty and peacefulness of nature has a unique power to automatically lift your spirits and inspire you. Add a heart-pumping walk to all that and you have the magic potion for feeling better, happier, and more energetic.

Walk the trail for fifteen minutes; then turn around and come back for a complete thirty-minute efficient workout. Of course, if you're going to the effort and can spare the time, go for a sixty- to ninety-minute nature walk. Take a friend or family member to keep you going at a steady pace and to help protect your safety. Be sure to pack a water bottle and drink often. As you walk, try to take the time to notice and appreciate the beauty of your surroundings.

How'd You Do? Count Your Whole Grains

Pop quiz: Think about everything you ate yesterday. I want you to add up how many servings of whole grains you ate throughout the day. Here's what counts as a serving:

- 1 slice 100-percent whole-wheat bread
- ½ whole-wheat bagel or small oat bran muffin
- ½ cup cooked whole-wheat pasta, brown rice, barley, bulgur, or wild rice
- 1 cup cooked oatmeal
- 1 cup high-fiber cereal (or whole-grain cereal with three or more grams of fiber per serving)
- 3 cups plain popcorn
- 1 whole-wheat tortilla

How did you do? You should eat three ounces (or three servings from the above list) of whole grains each day. If you didn't quite make three servings, do better today. Set a goal to eat at least three servings of *real* whole-grain foods. Watch out for sugary cereals and even cookies that claim "whole-grain" on the label. It's too good to be true. Stick to the list above for the most healthful whole grains.

TIP #168

Your Time to Shine

Make an appointment tonight to participate in a recreational activity. It can be something you've done before, "always wanted to but never tried" before, or something you do all the time. It's always more fun if you invite family members and/or friends to participate as well. Try a game of tennis, racquetball, swimming a few laps (make it a race), a game of softball, soccer, or flag football. There are many more—think about something you enjoy, or want to try, and go for it.

Make the arrangements right now. If you commit to it now, you'll actually have a chance of following through with it. You might find a new sport you enjoy and better yet, you may find yourself feeling stronger and more confident as you become more physically fit.

Comfortable Clothes to the Rescue—See Ya, Spandex!

For today's workout, wear your most comfortable clothing. If you work out at a gym, there's a higher probability that you may cave in and wear uncomfortable clothing that can be too tight or restrictive. I've worked in a gym for over ten years, and you know what? Nobody cares what anybody else is wearing—or doing for that matter. Most everyone in a health club is there to get healthier, stronger, or lose weight—sacrificing that valuable time to take care of themselves, not to observe others.

If you work out in your home, make sure the clothing is breathable as well as comfortable. It can be your pajamas, an old T-shirt—whatever makes you feel liberated and confident. Tight-fitting clothing can make you feel like you are overweight. Wearing such clothing is not a positive experience and can cause you to miss out on a great workout, as your mind stays distracted by how horribly your clothes fit or how uncomfortable they make you feel. Don't allow your workout time to become a negative experience because of a clothing choice. Put on something comfortable and get moving!

Broaden Your Taste Buds: Try a New Fruit Today

Apples and bananas. They are so easy, so well-liked, and so widely accessible. Of course they're healthy—but what about the many other kinds of fruits on the market today. If you tend to eat the same kinds of fruits day after day, take a stand today and try a new fruit you've never tried before. Variety is a crucial constituent of healthy living—we absolutely get more of the vital nutrients our bodies need by practicing variety.

Try one of these fruits today:

• Pomegranate	• Starfruit	• Kiwi
• Asian pear	• Passion fruit	• Fig
• Mango	• Blackberries	• Guava
• Papaya	• Boysenberries	• Kumquat

There are many more fruits from which you can choose. Check out the wide variety of fruit available in the produce section of your grocery store. If you aren't sure how to prepare or eat a certain fruit, do a quick search at www.about.com on the fruit of your choice or check out the handy recipe cards located next to the fruit in the produce section.

Tranquil Meditation Made Easy

Try some meditation today. In as little as ten minutes you can reduce anxiety, depression, moodiness, and stress. In addition, meditation puts your mind in the proper place to help you grow and progress on both a spiritual and a physical level.

Sit down on the floor; bend your knees out and bring your ankles close together in front of your hips. Rest your right hand on your right knee and your left hand on your left knee. Straighten your back and pull your belly button in toward your spine. Bring your shoulders down and back (as though you were trying to touch your shoulder blades together) and slightly lift your chin so that your eyes are looking straight forward. Now, close your eyes and start to breathe in and out in a slow controlled manner. Inhale *through the nose* deep into the lungs for two counts ("one one-thousand, two one-thousand") and exhale *out through the mouth* for two counts.

Sit in peace and quiet for ten minutes. Keep your abs contracted, your back straight, and your shoulders down. Focus on your breath and only your breath for the entire time.

Rethinking the Clean Plate Club

It's sad and unfortunate that there are starving people in this world. It's even more unfortunate, however, that because we have an overflowing food supply we somehow feel that we are helping with the starvation problem by "not wasting our food." It isn't good for our health, and it certainly doesn't help other people suffering from starvation.

Today, eat *until you are satisfied* and not *until your plate is clean*. Pay close attention to how you feel—try not to push yourself past the "satisfied" point. It's okay to push eating a few more bites of fruits, vegetables, whole grains, and low-fat dairy or soy—we don't get enough of those foods. But excess amounts of all the other stuff—starchy side dishes such as potatoes, white rice, refined pastas, meats, sweets, and treats—can be saved for later or thrown away. We eat too much of those foods. Cancel your membership to the Clean Plate Club and reclaim your health by feeding your body what it needs, and not more.

TIP #173

The Food You Don't Want to Eat in an Airport

If you are bustling through a busy airport today, make sure you *don't* stop for one of those gigantic hot cinnamon rolls. Those huge bakery items often sport 650 to 1000 calories and 30 to 40 grams of gunk (fat) for your arteries. It's a bummer, I know, but the delicate pastries, ice cream, and fresh-baked cookies sold in an airport don't make for the most healthy snacks. Your body is precious and you want to take care of it— always remember that. Treat your body right and try one of these more healthy foods at the airport instead:

- Pretzels (plain, without butter or dips)
- Apples or bananas
- Mixed nuts (eat only two handfuls)
- Dried fruit
- Small sandwich (on wheat bread, if possible)
- Sugar-free frozen yogurt
- Single hamburger or breakfast sandwich *without* cheese
- Fruit smoothie (small size only!)
- One-quarter to one-half of a sweet treat (share with a friend if you must indulge)

How Much Exercise Do I Really Need?

The new government recommendations for physical activity are bold when you consider the fact that 68 percent of us fail to get the minimum thirty minutes per day on most days of the week. But the recommendations are spot on—they tell us what we need desperately.

What will you do today? In an ideal world, here's the amount of exercise you should do*:

- *Thirty minutes* of moderate intensity exercise on most days of the week can reduce the risk of chronic disease in adulthood.
- *Sixty minutes* of moderate intensity exercise on most days of the week can manage body weight and prevent gradual, unhealthy body weight gain in adulthood.
- *Sixty to ninety minutes* of moderate intensity exercise on most days of the week can sustain weight loss in adulthood.

A "moderate intensity" level of exercise is different for everyone. Moderate to a runner might be six miles per hour, whereas moderate to an elderly person might be two miles per hour. Moderate intensity should feel challenging but comfortable. You should be able to speak a few words at a time and breathe in a controlled manner as you exercise.

Dietary Guidelines for Americans 2005 (U.S. Department of Health and Human Services and the U.S. Department of Agriculture), chapter 4.

A Better Birthday Party

Have you got a birthday party to attend today? If it's not your own birthday, resolve right now to practice moderation. (If it is your own birthday, enjoy the once-a-year day and eat what you want!) Take a moment to seriously think about how you can enjoy the fun *without overdoing all the food.* Here are a few ideas:

- Cut back on the starchy foods served during the meal (so you can enjoy the cake!). Breadsticks, potatoes, and rolls, along with macaroni, potato, or fruit salads covered in whipped topping are all foods you should eat less of (half-sized portions down to none at all) so you can save room for the birthday dessert.
- Instead of the starchy foods, eat fresh fruit, raw veggies, or some leafy greens with low-fat dressing.
- Enjoy a "sensible" serving of cake and ice cream. A two-inch square of chocolate cake and a small one-half cup serving of ice cream has 550 calories, 31 grams of fat, and 45 grams of sugar (11 teaspoons). So don't go for seconds.

New Exercise Move: The Bridge

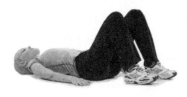

Try doing the bridge exercise today. It requires no equipment and works to strengthen your glutes, lower back, abdominals, and obliques.

Lie down on your back on the floor. Bend your knees, place your feet flat on the floor about twelve inches from your hips, and point your toes forward. Place your hands straight at your sides, near your hips, with your palms flat on the floor. Now, dig your weight into your heels and contract your glutes. Keeping that contraction, push your hips up toward the ceiling until your knees, hips, and shoulders are in a straight diagonal line. Then slowly lower your hips back down to the floor. Exhale through your mouth as you lift; inhale through your nose as you lower.

Perform fifteen to twenty-five reps at a 1–1–1 tempo (1 second up, 1 second hold at the top, and 1 second down).

Perform another fifteen to twenty-five reps at a 2–2–2 tempo (2 seconds up, 2 second hold, and 2 seconds down).

Perform the most reps you can in good form. Always listen to your body and work at your own pace.

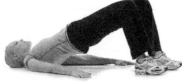

Oversized Starches, Be Gone

Nobody in this country is suffering from eating supersized portions of steamed broccoli or juicy watermelon. The real supersize offenders are the starchy foods, salty snacks, and sweet treats. So today make the effort to find out how big your "normal" portions are. Focus on the starchy foods. If you eat pasta, rice, or potatoes, measure the amount you dish up before you eat it. Sometimes we are a little naïve—we tend to *underestimate* the amount of food we dish up and *overestimate* the amount of activity we perform on a daily basis. It's human nature. So be open-minded; it's possible you are dishing up two to three cups (or two to three times the recommended portion size) of pasta, rice, or potatoes.

If you are eating one of these foods in a restaurant today, you have a 100-percent guarantee that you'll be served a double, triple, or even quadruple serving of starchy food. So plan to eat one-half of what they serve and take the rest home for later.

How to Find the Best Workout Music

It's undisputed. Music adds much-needed motivation to keep workouts exciting and fun. But in order to find seriously beneficial workout music, you need to know the beats per minute (or "BPMs"). BPMs are the number of beats that occur in sixty seconds—essentially the "pace" of the music. Check out your favorite music today; count the number of beats you hear in fifteen seconds and multiply by four (or count the number of beats you hear in sixty seconds). If you use iTunes, you can view the BPMs for each song by right-clicking the menu bar.

Find a BPM that matches your preferred activity, so you can try to step or move on every beat—this keeps your pace consistent, steady, and effective. BPMs are the perfect, built-in pacesetter. You'll get more out of your workout and a healthier return for your time.

115 BPM
- Slow walking
- Strength training

125 BPM
- Elliptical training
- Stair climbing
- Walking (3–4 mph)

135 BPM
- Power/fitness walking (4–4.5 mph)
- Moderate cycling (60–70 rpm)

145 BPM
- Jogging (5–6 mph)
- Fast cycling (75–80 rpm)

On Vacation? Make Time for Exercise

If you're on vacation, one thing is certain: you're likely to eat more than usual. And if you're on one of those relaxing vacations (*not* Disneyland, which was our last vacation spot), you likely have more time on your hands. Combine these factors and you've got a very convincing reason to exercise. Make time for some activity while you vacation away. You're not wasting your vacation time by spending thirty minutes to rejuvenate your day. If you can make it a group effort, even better; you still get to enjoy time together along with some great scenery. Exercise can improve your mood and your energy level, making your vacation all the better. Try one of these today:

- Go on a scenic hike.
- Rent bikes and go for a scenic bike ride.
- Go for a fast walk on the beach.
- Visit the local health club.
- Try out the hotel fitness center.
- March or jog in place (or do jumping jacks) while you watch the morning news.
- Try the no-equipment strength workout found in Tip #105.

Staying Committed to Your Goals: Say It Out Loud!

If you're having one of those days—you know, wondering why you are trying so hard to get healthy and not feeling a worthwhile benefit just yet—try talking to a family member or friend about why you want to be healthier. Tell them what you want and why it's been so hard to stick with it lately. Saying it out loud reinforces your intentions and helps you stick to your mental commitments. Really.

Actually saying the words out loud, like: "I want to have the strength to go on a hike with my children" or "I want to feel better and be a happier person—and I know exercise helps me do that, but sometimes I just can't get out of bed" can make you realize that (1) it's something you *really* want and (2) maybe your barriers (like being too busy, too tired, etc.) can be overcome if you rethink your priorities and recommit to feeling healthy and strong. When you are healthy, you can take better care of those around you—and enjoy doing it!

Work In, Out, and Around the Fat-Burning Zone

It's often said that you have to work out for at least thirty minutes at a specific intensity level to "burn fat." But really, in a world where inactivity is rampant, we simply need to get moving—in any way possible! People get so caught up with staying in that "moderate-intensity fat-burning zone" that they miss out on pushing themselves a bit harder to really improve their fitness level. Strength training is stop and go, so it's not a typical fat-burning zone either. But strength training builds lean calorie-burning muscle, which then boosts your metabolic rate—which is definitely worth jumping out of that fat-burn zone.

So shake up your workouts. It's okay to work at a comfortable pace for a longer period of time one day (about sixty minutes), a moderate pace another day (about thirty to forty minutes), and a challenging pace a third day (about twenty to thirty minutes). Doing so keeps your body from adapting to the same routine.

Try working at a new intensity level today; work at a *slower pace* for a longer period of time or a *harder pace* for a shorter period of time.

Surviving the Steak House

If you're visiting a steak restaurant sometime today or in the near future, try to follow these healthier recommendations to keep your next steakhouse visit in the "I don't have to spend four hours on the treadmill" category.

- Share your entrée with a friend. Split the enormous slab of meat in two and order an extra side (veggies would be good!) to make two filling meals.
- Don't order "loaded baked potatoes." Eat a baked potato with one topping only—or better yet, with a little salt and pepper (your meat will have plenty of fat, so you don't need fat on your potato, too). If you order mashed potatoes, order the gravy on the side.
- Order a salad topped with chunks of fresh vegetables. It can be your appetizer or, even better, your side dish to the meat. Order the dressing on the side.
- Remember *sirloin*, the leanest cut of red meat. It still has about fifteen grams of fat in a twelve-ounce steak, but it is the lowest in fat overall. Porterhouse, T-bone, New York strip, and prime rib all have more than double that amount of fat.

No Time for Breakfast?

If you have no time to pour a bowl of cereal, let alone cook a hot breakfast before racing out the door, try one of these convenient, easy, and healthy breakfast options:

Grab-n-Go Breakfast Options from Home
- All-Bran Cereal Bites (these are very tasty!)
- All-Bran Granola Bars
- Light vanilla yogurt and a banana
- String cheese and an apple
- Dry Kashi or any high-fiber cereal (in a plastic bag)
- Cottage cheese (single-serving container)
- One handful of nuts and one large handful of grapes
- Dry packets of plain instant oatmeal (you can even cook it when you get to the office)

Drive-thru Breakfast Options
- Yogurt and fruit
- An egg and cheese English muffin (one meat only, no croissants)
- A whole-wheat bagel with peanut butter
- Scrambled eggs and fruit

Easy Spaghetti Dinners Made Healthier

Spaghetti is one of the all-time easiest dinners. Brown some lean hamburger, boil a few noodles, dump a bottle of spaghetti sauce over it, and call it good. Right? Not quite. With a few modifications, this meal can be improved a great deal. It can be made into something really exquisite, because it's healthy *and* easy. And that means a lot in today's busy times.

For tonight's dinner, use whole-wheat spaghetti instead of the usual refined spaghetti. Go easy on the bottled spaghetti sauce to cut back on sodium (spaghetti sauce is okay because it's a very rich source of the antioxidant lycopene). Skip the sliced white or French bread with garlic spread and try serving a steamed vegetable and a fresh green salad instead. Add some fruit to sweeten the meal, like berries with a sprinkle of sugar or one cup cubed cantaloupe and watermelon.

You'll get three times the fiber thanks to the whole-wheat noodles, and you'll save yourself a good 200 calories and 10 grams of fat just by cutting out the garlic bread. Those are simple things that make a big difference.

The Talk Test

Test yourself. Work out at your "normal" intensity level for at least thirty minutes today. At fifteen minutes—the peak of your workout session— try the "talk test." See how much you can talk.

Are you working and breathing so hard that you can barely utter a word? If so, you are likely in the anaerobic, "without oxygen" zone. It's fine to work in this zone once in a while, but make sure you don't feel light-headed or faint. You should still feel in control of your breathing.

If you can't talk at all, you are definitely working too hard and should drop your intensity down to a level in which you can speak and control your breathing.

If you can carry on full conversations and tell long elaborate stories, you are not working hard enough! So step it up! (Or plan to stay at that intensity level for *at least* one hour.) If you are going to take the time to exercise, make sure you work at a level that is going to make a difference in your health.

TIP #186

Don't Waste Calories on Frozen Chocolate

It's a cold, hard fact. Frozen chocolate just doesn't have the delicious flavor of room temperature or warm chocolate. Yet ice cream filled with chocolate chunks or candy bar bits is growing ever more popular, and shakes crowded with endless toppings and mix-ins are popping up in fast-food outlets and ice cream shops across the nation. Those chocolate chunks may seem small and insignificant, but the reality is that every "scoop" of candy bar chunks adds about 150 calories and 5 grams of fat. So a regular shake with two types of chocolate "mix-ins" has an extra 300 calories and 10 grams of fat—I'd call that a pretty significant contribution to the calorie mix.

My rule is simple: if you can't taste it, don't eat it! Don't torment yourself by wasting your calories on the extra stuff added to sweeten a food that is already plenty sweet (ice cream isn't bland in flavor, by any means). Enjoy the ice cream plain, or with fruit, a few nuts, or a drizzle of chocolate topping. Save your calories for foods you can fully taste, enjoy, and savor.

On Second Thought . . .

Keep track of everything you do today. Write down what you do and approximately what time you do it. For example:

6:30 A.M. Scripture study
7:00 A.M. Cook breakfast
7:30 A.M. Wash dishes
8:00 A.M. Start laundry and pick up house
9:00 A.M. Drive kids to swimming lessons
And so forth . . .

Keeping a log of your "time use" for *just one day* will help you identify potential windows of opportunity to find some time for yourself—to exercise, to eat a healthy snack, or to take a quiet moment to de-stress. You may have to swap an activity or steal ten minutes here and there.

This time-use log will also help you realize the sheer amount of time you likely spend serving and doing good works for others. This is important. We are so hard on ourselves, beating ourselves up because we "didn't get to" this or that. Give credit where credit is due! You work hard; it's okay *and necessary* to take a few moments for yourself. This helps you find the strength to do the things you were sent here to do.

To Eat Less, Keep That Minty Clean Feeling

Are you having a craving for something sweet? Does it happen every day about the same time? Try this: brush your teeth, put a stick of gum in your mouth, or start sipping water from a water bottle or glass.

This little trick works for me all the time. If I've already eaten breakfast and find myself looking through the cupboards for everything and anything with sugar or chocolate, I quickly go and brush my teeth and start drinking some water. It really works! Sugar just doesn't taste as good after you brush your teeth. And after going to the effort of brushing, you'll have at least a little bit of time where you want to keep that nice clean feeling before you fill your teeth with some gritty sugar. You can even keep a toothbrush in your desk drawer if you experience food temptations while you are at the office.

Walking with Weights?

Do you wonder if you should wear ankle weights while walking? Maybe hold some hand weights while you pump your arms?

The truth is that it's possible that walking with light weights flailing around can do more harm than good; because the weight is not centered (like in the trunk area of your body), you are adding unnecessary stress to your joints and ligaments. In addition, the weight really isn't heavy enough to increase your calorie burn to a significant level. If you want to try weighted walking, wear a weight vest—something that is centered over your chest, back, and abdominals.

The ideal situation? Make your walk fast and quick, pump those arms, and walk with short, quick steps. Then perform strength training (with deliberate, controlled movements) at a separate time; working all the major muscles of your body (like legs, chest, back, shoulders, arms, and abdominals) two to four days a week for thirty to sixty minutes.